Stammering, Its Cause and Cure

Benjamin Nathaniel Bogue

Contents

STAMMERING,
ITS CAUSE AND CURE

BY

Benjamin Nathaniel Bogue

TO MY MOTHER

That wonderful woman whose unflagging courage held me to a task
that I never could have completed alone and who when all others
failed, stood by me, encouraged me and pointed out the heights where
lay success--this volume is dedicated

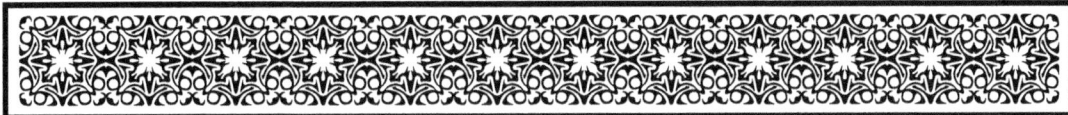

PREFACE

Considerably more than a third of a century has elapsed since I purchased my first book on stammering. I still have that quaint little book made up in its typically English style with small pages, small type and yellow paper back--the work of an English author whose obtuse and half-baked theories certainly lent no clarity to the stammerer's understanding of his trouble. Since that first purchase my library of books on stammering has grown until it is perhaps the largest individual collection in the world. I have read these books--many of them several times, pondered over the obscurities in some, smiled at the absurdities in others and benefited by the truths in a few. Yet, with all their profound explanations of theories and their verbose defense of hopelessly unscientific methods, the stammerer would be disappointed indeed, should he attempt to find in the entire collection a practical and understandable discussion of his trouble.

This insufficiency of existing books on stammering has encouraged me to bring out the present volume. It is needed. I know this-- because I spent almost twenty years of my life in a well-nigh futile search for the very knowledge herein revealed. I haunted the libraries, was a familiar figure in book stores and a frequent visitor to the second-hand dealer. Yet these efforts brought me comparatively little--not one-tenth the information that this book contains.

Perhaps it is but a colossal conceit that prompts me to offer this volume to those who stutter and stammer as I did. Yet, I cannot but believe that almost twenty years' personal experience as a stammerer plus more than twenty-eight years' experience in curing speech disorders has supplied me with an intensely practical, valuable and worth-while knowledge on which to base this book.

After having stammered for twenty years you have pretty well run the whole gamut of mockery, humiliation and failure. You understand the stammerer's feelings, his mental processes and his peculiarities.

And when you add to this more than a quarter of a century, every waking hour of which has been spent in alleviating the stammerer's difficulty--and successfully, too--you have a ground-work of first-hand information that tends toward facts instead of fiction and toward practice instead of theory.

These are my qualifications.

I have spent a life-time in studying stammering, stuttering and kindred speech defects. I have written this book out of the fullness of that experience--I might almost say out of my daily work. I have made no attempt at literary style or rhetorical excellence and while the work may be homely in expression the information it contains is definite and positive--and what is more important--it is authoritative.

I hope the reader will find the book useful--yes, and helpful. I hope he will find in it the way to Freedom of Speech--his birthright and the birthright of every man.

BENJAMIN NATHANIEL BOGUE
Indianapolis September, 1929

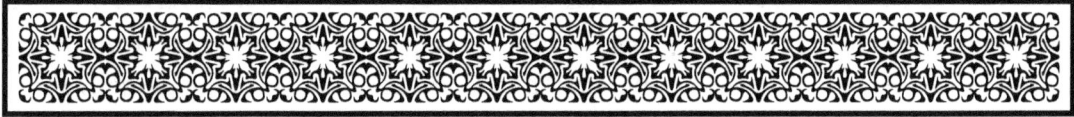

PART I
MY LIFE AS A STAMMERER

CHAPTER I
STARTING LIFE UNDER A HANDICAP

I was laughed at for nearly twenty years because I stammered. I found school a burden, college a practical impossibility and life a misery because of my affliction.

I was born in Wabash county, Indiana, and as far back as I can remember, there was never a time when I did not stammer or stutter. So far as I know, the halting utterance came with the first word I spoke and for almost twenty years this difficulty continued to dog me relentlessly.

When six years of age, I went to the little school house down the road, little realizing what I was to go through with there before I left.

Previous to the time I entered school, those around me were my family, my relatives and my friends--people who were very kind and considerate, who never spoke of my difficulty in my presence, and certainly never laughed at me.

At school, it was quite another matter. It was fun for the other boys to hear me speak and it was common pastime with them to get me to talk whenever possible. They would jibe and jeer--and then ask, "What did you say? Why don't you learn to talk English?" Their best entertainment was to tease and mock me until I became angry, taunt me when I did, and ridicule me at every turn.

It was not only in the school yard and going to and from school that I suffered--but also in class. When I got up to recite, what a spectacle I made, hesitating over every other word, stumbling along, gasping for breath, waiting while speech returned to me. And how they laughed at me--for then I was helpless to defend myself. True, my teachers tried to be kind to me, but that did not make me talk normally like other children, nor did it always prevent the others from laughing at me.

The reader can imagine my state of mind during these school days. I fairly hated even to start to school in the morning--not because I disliked to go to school, but because I was sure to meet some of my taunting comrades, sure to be humiliated and laughed at because I stammered. And having reached the school room I had to face the prospect of failing every time I stood up on my feet and tried to recite.

There were four things I looked forward to with positive dread-- the trip to school, the recitations in class, recess in the school yard and the trip home again. It makes me shudder even now to think of those days--the dread with which I left that home of mine every school day morning, the nervous strain, the torment and torture, and the constant fear of failure which never left me. Imagine my thoughts as I left parents and friends to face the ribald laughter of those who did not understand. I asked myself: "Well, what new disgrace today? Whom will I meet this morning? What will the teacher say when I stumble? How shall I get through recess? What is the easiest way home?"

These and a hundred other questions, born of nervousness and fear, I asked myself morning after morning. And day after day, as the hours dragged by, I would wonder, "Will this day NEVER end? Will I NEVER get out of this?"

Such was my life in school. And such is the daily life of thousands of boys and hundreds of girls--a life of dread, of constant fear, of endless worry and unceasing nervousness.

But, as I look back at the boys and girls who helped to make life miserable for me in school, I feel for them only kindness. I bear no malice. They did no more than their fathers and mothers, many of them, would have done. They little realized what they were doing. They had no intention to do me personal injury, though there is no question in my mind but that they made my trouble worse. They did not know how terribly they were punishing me. They saw in my affliction only fun, while I saw in it--only misery.

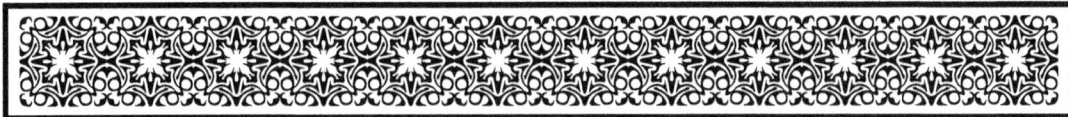

CHAPTER II
MY FIRST ATTEMPT TO BE CURED

I can remember very clearly the positive fear which always accompanied a visit to our friends or neighbors, or the advent of visitors at my home. Many a time I did not have what I desired to eat because I was afraid to ask for it. When I did ask, every eye was turned on me, and the looks of the strangers, with now and then a half-suppressed smile, worked me up to a nervous state that was almost hysterical, causing me to stutter worse than at any other time.

At one time--I do not remember what the occasion was--a number of people had come to visit us. A large table had been set and loaded with good things. We sat down, the many dishes were passed around the table, as was the custom at our home, and I said not a word. But before long the first helping was gone--a hungry boy soon cleans his plate--and I was about to ask for more when I bethought myself. "Please pass--" I could never do it--"p" was one of the hard sounds for me. "Please pass--" No, I couldn't do it. So busying myself with the things that were near at hand and helping myself to those things which came my way, I made out the meal--but I got up from the table hungry and with a deeper consciousness of the awfulness of my affliction. Slowly it began to dawn on me that as long as I stammered I was doomed to do without much of the world's goods. I began to see that although I might for a time sit at the World's Table of Good Things in Life I could hope to have little save that which someone passed on to me gratuitously.

As long as I was at home with my parents, life went along fairly well. They understood my difficulty, they sympathized with me, and they looked at my trouble in the same light as myself--as an affliction much to be regretted. At home I was not required to do anything which would embarrass me or cause me to become highly excited because of my straining to talk, but on the other hand I was permitted to do things which I could do well, without talking to any one.

The time was coming, however, when it would be "Sink or Swim" for me, since it would not be many years until a sense of duty, if nothing else, would send me out to make my own way. This time comes to all boys. It was soon to be MY task to face the world--to make a living for myself. And this was a thing which, strangely enough for a boy of my age, I began to think about. I had some experience in meeting people and in trying to transact some of the minor business connected with our farm and I found out that I had no chance along that line as long as I stammered.

And yet it seemed as if I was to be compelled to continue to stammer the rest of my life, for my condition was getting worse every day. This was very clear to me--and very plain to my parents. They were anxious to do something for me and do it quickly, so they called in a skilled physician. They told him about my trouble. He gave me a cursory examination and decided that my stuttering was caused by nervousness, and gave me some very distasteful medicine, which I was compelled to take three times a day. This medicine did me no good. I took it for five years, but there was no progress made toward curing my stuttering. The reason was simple. Stuttering cannot be cured by bitter medicine. The physician was using the wrong method. He was treating the effect and not the cause. He was of the opinion that it was the nervousness that caused my stuttering, whereas the fact of the matter was, it was my stuttering that caused the nervousness.

I do not blame this physician in the least because of his failure, for he was not an expert on the subject of speech defects. While he was a medical man of known ability, he had not made a study of speech disorders and knew practically nothing about either the cause or cure of stammering or stuttering. Even today, prominent medical men will tell you that their profession has given little or no attention to defects of speech and take little interest in such cases.

Some time later, after the physician had failed to benefit me, a traveling medicine man came to our community, set up his tent, and stayed for a week. Of course, like all traveling medicine men, his remedies were cure-alls. One night in making his talk before the crowd, he mentioned the fact that his wonderful concoction, taken with the pamphlet that he would furnish, both for the sum of one dollar, would cure stammering. I didn't have the dollar, so I did not buy. But the next day I went back, and I took the dollar along. He got my dollar, and I still have the book.

Of course, I received no benefit whatever. I later came to the conclusion that the medicine man had been in the neighborhood long enough to have pointed out to him "BEN BOGUE'S BOY WHO STUTTERS" (as I was known) and had decided that when I was in his audience a hint or two on the virtues of his wonderful remedy in cases of stammering, would be sufficient to extract a dollar from me for a tryout.

These experiences, however, were valuable to me, even though they were costly, for they taught me a badly-needed lesson, to wit: That drugs and medicines are not a cure for stammering.

Many of the people who came in contact with me, and those who talked the matter over with my parents, said that I would outgrow the trouble. "All that is necessary," remarked one man, "is for him to forget that he stammers, and the trouble will be gone."

This was a rather foolish suggestion and simply proved how little the man knew about the subject. In the first place, a stammerer cannot forget his difficulty--who can say that he would be cured if he did? You might as well say to a man holding a hot poker, "If you will only forget that the poker is hot, it will be cool." It takes something more than forgetfulness to cure stammering.

The belief held by both my parents and myself that I would outgrow my difficulty was one of the gravest mistakes we ever made. Had I followed the advice of others who believed in the outgrowing theory it eventually would have caused me to become a confirmed stammerer, entirely beyond hope of cure.

Today, as a result of twenty-eight years' daily contact with stammerers, I know that stammering cannot be outgrown. The man who suggests that it is possible to cure stammering by outgrowing it is doing a great injustice to the stammerer, because he is giving him a false hope--in fact the most futile hope that any stammerer ever had. I wish I could paint in the sky, in letters of fire, the truth that "Stammering cannot be outgrown," because this, of all things, is the most frequent pitfall of the stammerer, his greatest delusion and one of the most prolific causes of continued suffering. I know whereof I speak, because I tried it myself. I know how many different people held up to me the hope that I would outgrow it.

My father offered me a valuable shotgun if I would stop stammering. My mother offered me money, a watch and a horse and buggy. These inducements made me strain every nerve to stop my imperfect utterance, but all to no avail. At this time I knew nothing of the underlying principles of speech and any effort which I made to stop my stammering was merely a crude, misdirected attempt which naturally had no chances for success.

I learned that prizes will never cure stammering. I found out too, something I have never since forgotten: that the man, woman or child who stammers needs no inducement to cause him to desire to be cured, because the change from his condition as a stammerer to that of a nonstammerer is of more inducement to the sufferer than all the money you could offer him. I have never yet seen a man, woman or child who wanted to stammer or stutter.

The offer of prizes doing no good, I took long trips to get my mind off the affliction. I did everything in my power, worked almost day and night, exerted every effort I could command--it was all in vain.

The idea that I would finally outgrow my difficulty was strengthened in the minds of my parents and friends by the fact that there were times when my impediment seemed almost to disappear, but to our surprise and disappointment, it always came back again, each time in a more aggravated form; each time with a stronger hold upon me than ever before.

I found out, then, one of the fundamental characteristics of stammering--its intermittent tendency. In other words, I discovered that a partial relief from the difficulty was one of the true symptoms of the malady. And I learned further that this relief is only temporary and not what we first thought it to be, viz: a sign that the disorder was leaving.

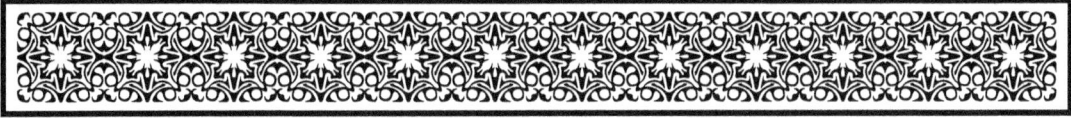

CHAPTER III
MY SEARCH CONTINUES

My parents' efforts to have me cured, however, did not cease with my visit to the medicine man. We were still looking for something that would bring relief. My teacher, Miss Cora Critchlow, handed me an advertisement one day, telling me of a man who claimed to be able to cure stammering by mail. In the hope that I would get some good from the treatment, my parents sent this mail order man a large sum of money. In return for this I was furnished with instructions to do a number of useless things, such as holding toothpicks between my teeth, talking through my nose, whistling before I spoke a word, and many other foolish things. It was at this time that I learned once and for all, the imprudence of throwing money away on these mail order "cures," so-called, and I made up my mind to bother no more with this man and his kind.

So far as the mail order instructions were concerned, they were crude and unscientific--merely a hodge-podge of pseudo-technical phraseology and crass ignorance--a meaningless jargon scarcely intelligible to the most highly educated, and practically impossible of interpretation by the average stammerer who was supposed to follow the course. Even after I had, by persistent effort, interpreted the instructions and followed them closely for many months, there was not a sign of the slightest relief from my trouble. It was evident to me even then that I could never cure myself by following a mail cure.

Today, after twenty-eight years of experience in the cure of stammering, I can say with full authority, that stammering cannot be successfully treated by mail. The very nature of the difficulty, as well as the method of treatment, make it impossible to put the instructions into print or to have the stammerer follow out the method from a printed sheet.

As I approached manhood, my impediment began to get worse. My stuttering changed to stammering. Instead of rapidly repeating syllables or words, I was unable to begin a word. I stood transfixed, my limbs drawing themselves into all kinds of unnatural positions. There were violent spasmodic movements of the head, and contractions of my whole body. The muscles of my throat would swell, affecting the respiratory organs, and causing a curious barking sound. When I finally got started, I would utter the first part of the sentence slowly, gradually increase the speed, and make a rush toward the end.

At other times, when attempting to speak, my lips would pucker up, firmly set together, and I would be unable to separate them, until my breath was exhausted. Then I would gasp for more breath, struggling with the words I desired to speak, until the veins of my forehead would swell, my face would become red, and I would sink back, wholly unable to express myself, and usually being obliged to resort to writing.

These paroxysms left me extremely nervous and in a seriously weakened condition. After one of these attacks, the cold perspiration would break out on my forehead in great beads and I would sink into the nearest chair, where I would be compelled to remain until I had regained my strength.

My affliction was taking all my energy, sapping my strength, deadening my mental faculties, and placing me at a hopeless disadvantage in every way. I could do nothing that other people did. I appeared unnatural. I was nervous, irritable, despondent. This despondency now brought about a peculiar condition. I began to believe that everyone was more or less an enemy of mine. And still worse, I came to believe that I was an enemy of myself, which feeling threw me into despair, the depths of which I do not wish to recall, even now.

I was not only miserably unhappy myself, I made everyone else around me unhappy, although I did it, not intentionally, but because my affliction had caused me to lose control of myself.

In this condition, my nerves were strained to the breaking point all day long, and many a night I can remember crying myself to sleep--crying purely to relieve that stored-up nervous tension, and f ailing off to sleep as a result of exhaustion.

As I said before, there were periods of grace when the trouble seemed almost to vanish and I would be delighted to believe that perhaps it was gone forever--happy hope! But it was but a delusion, a mirage in the distance, a new road to lead me astray. The affliction always returned, as every stammerer knows--returned worse than before. All the hopes that I would outgrow my trouble, were found to be false hopes. For me, there was no such thing as outgrowing it and I have since discovered that after the age of six only one-fifth of one per cent. ever outgrow the trouble.

Another thing which I always thought peculiar when I was a stammerer was the fact that I had practically no difficulty in talking to animals when I was alone with them. I remember very well that we had a large bulldog called Jim, which I was very fond of. I used to believe that Jim understood my troubles better than any friend I had, unless it was Old Sol, our family driving horse.

Jim used to go with me on all my jaunts--I could talk to him by the hour and never stammer a word. And Old Sol--well, when everything seemed to be going against me, I used to go out and talk things over with Old Sol. Somehow he seemed to understand--he used to whinney softly and rub his nose against my shoulder as if to say, "I understand, Bennie, I understand!"

Somehow my father had discovered this peculiarity of my affliction--that is, my ability to talk to animals or when alone. Something suggested to him that my stammering could be cured, if I could be kept by myself for several weeks. With this thought in mind, he suggested that I go on a hunting and fishing trip in the wilds of the northwest, taking no guide, no companion of any sort, so that there would be no necessity of my speaking to any human being while I was gone.

My father's idea was that if my vocal organs had a complete rest, I would be restored to perfect speech. As I afterwards proved to my own satisfaction by actual trial, this idea was entirely wrong. You can not hope to restore the proper action of your vocal organs by ceasing to use them. The proper functioning of any bodily organ is the result, not of ceasing to use it at all, but rather of using it correctly.

This can be very easily proved to the satisfaction of any one. Take the case of the small boy who boasts of his muscle. He is conscious of an increasing strength in the muscles of his arm not because he has failed to use these muscles but because he has used them continually, causing a faster-than-ordinary development.

You can readily imagine that I looked forward to my "vacation" with keen anticipation, for I had never been up in the northwest and I was full of stories I had read and ideas I had formed of its wonders.

The trip, lasting two weeks, did me scarcely any good at all. The most I can say for it is that it quieted my nerves and put me in somewhat better physical condition, which a couple of weeks in the outdoor country would do for any growing boy.

But this trip did not cure my stammering, nor did it tend to alleviate the intensity of the trouble in the least, save through a lessened nervous state for a few days. Today, after twenty-eight years' experience, I know that it would be just as sensible to say that a wagon stuck in the soft mud would get out by "resting" there as it is to say that stammering can be eradicated by allowing the vocal organs to rest through disuse.

Shortly after my return from the trip to the northwest, my father died, with the result that our household was, for a time, very much broken up. For a while, at least, my stammering, though not forgotten, did not receive a great deal of attention, for there were many other things to think about.

The summer following my father's death, however, I began again my so-far fruitless search for a cure for my stammering, this time placing myself under the care and instruction of a man claiming to be "The World's Greatest Specialist in the Cure of Stammering." He may have been the world's greatest specialist, but not in the cure of stammering. He did succeed, however, by the use of his absurd methods, in putting me through a course that resulted in the membrane and lining of my throat and vocal organs becoming irritated and inflamed to such an extent that I was compelled to undergo treatment for a throat affection that threatened to be as serious as the stammering itself. I tried everything that came to my attention--first one thing and then another--but without results. Still I refused to be discouraged. I kept on and on, my mother constantly encouraging and reassuring me. And you will later see that I found a method that cured me.

There are always those who stand idly about and say, "It can't be done!" Such people as these laughed at Fulton with his steamboat, they laughed at Stephenson and his steam locomotive, they laughed at Wright and the airplane.

They say, "It can't be done"--but it is done, nevertheless.

I turned a deaf ear to the people who tried to convince me that it couldn't be done. I had a firm belief in that old adage, "Where there is a will there is a way," and I made another of my own, which said, "I will FIND a way or MAKE one!"

And I did!

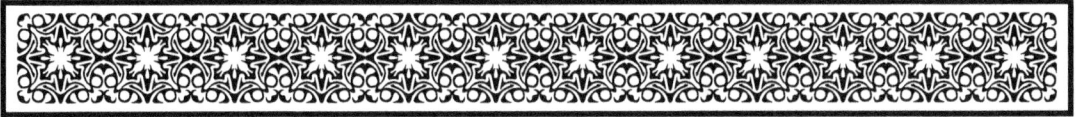

CHAPTER IV
A STAMMERER HUNTS A JOB

After recovering from my sad experiment with the "Wonderful Specialist," I did not want to go home and listen to the Anvil Chorus of "It Can't Be Done!" and "I Told You So!" I had no desire to be the object of laughter as well as pity. So I tried to get a job in that same city. I went from office to office--but nobody had a job for a man who stammered.

Finally I did land a job, however, such as it was. My duties were to operate the elevator in a hotel. How I managed to get that job, I often wonder now, for nobody on whom I called had any place for a boy or man who stammered. I thought it would be easy to find a job where I wouldn't need to talk, but when I started out to look for this job, I found it wasn't so easy after all. Almost any job requires a man who can talk. This I had learned in my own search for a place. But somehow or other, I managed to get that job as elevator boy in a hotel.

For the work as elevator boy I was paid three dollars a week. Wasn't that great pay for a man grown? But that's what I got.

That is, I got it for a little while, until I lost my job. For lose it I did before very long. I found out that I couldn't do much with even an elevator boy's job at three dollars a week unless I could talk. My employer found it out, too, and then he found somebody who could take my place--a boy who could answer when spoken to.

Well, here I was out of a job again. I am afraid I came pretty near being discouraged about that time. Things looked pretty hopeless for me--it was mighty hard work to get a job and the place didn't last long after I had gotten it.

But, nevertheless, the only thing to do was to try again. I started the search all over again. I tried first one place and then another. One man wanted me to start out as a salesman. He showed me how I could make more money than I had ever made in my life--convinced me that I could make it. Then I started to tell my part of the story--but I didn't get very far before he discovered that I was a stammerer. That was enough for him--with a gesture of hopelessness, he turned to his desk. "You'll never do, young man, you'll never do. You can't even talk!" And the worst of it was that he was right.

I once thought I had landed a job as stock chaser in a factory, but here, too, stammering barred the way, for they told me that even the stock chaser had to be able to deliver verbal messages from one foreman to another. I didn't dare to try that.

Eventually, I drifted around to the Union News Company. They wanted a boy to sell newspapers on trams running out over the Grand Trunk Railway. I took the job--the last job in the world I should have expected to hold, because of all the places a newsboy's job is one where you need to have a voice and the ability to talk.

I hope no stammerer ever has a position that causes him as much humiliation and suffering as that job caused me. You can imagine what it meant to me to go up and down the aisles of the train, calling papers and every few moments finding out that I couldn't say what I started out to say and then go gasping and grunting down the aisle making all sorts of facial grimaces.

How the passengers laughed at me! And how they made fun of me and asked me all sorts of questions just to hear me try to talk. It almost made me wish I could never see a human being again, so keen was the suffering and so tense were my nerves as a result of this work.

I don't believe I ever did anything that kept me in a more frenzied mental state than this work of trying to sell newspapers --and it wasn't very long (as I had expected) until the manager found out my situation and gently let me out.

Then I gave up, all at once. Was I discouraged? Well, perhaps. But not exactly discouraged. Rather I saw the plain hopelessness of trying to get or hold a job in my condition. So I prepared to go home. I didn't want to do it, because I knew the neighbors and friends round about would be ready for me with, "I told you so" and "I knew it couldn't be done" and a lot of gratuitous information like that.

But I gave up, nevertheless, deeply disappointed to think that once again I had failed to be cured of stammering, yet all the while resolving just as firmly as ever that I would try again and that I would never give up hope as long as there remained anything for me to do.

And this rule I followed out, month after month and year after year, until in the end I was richly rewarded for my patience and persistence.

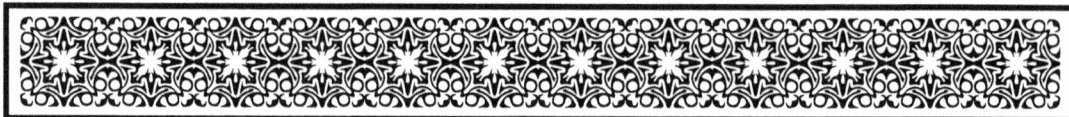

CHAPTER V
FURTHER FUTILE ATTEMPTS TO BE CURED

The next summer I decided to visit eastern institutions for the cure of stammering and determine if these could do any more for me than had already been done-which as the reader has seen, was practically nothing. I bought a ticket for Philadelphia, where I remained for some time, and where I gained more information of value than in all of my previous efforts combined.

I found in the Quaker City an old man who had made speech defects almost a life study. He knew more about the true principles of speech and the underlying fundamentals in the production of voice than all of the rest put together. He taught me these things, and gave me a solid foundation on which to build. True, he did not cure my stammering. But that was not because he failed to understand its cause, but merely because he had not worked out the correct method of removing the cause.

It was this man who first brought home to me the fact that principles of speech are constant, that they never change and that every person who talks normally follows out the same principles of speech, while every person who stutters or stammers violates these principles of speech. That is the basis of sound procedure for the cure of stammering and I must acknowledge my indebtedness to this sincere old gentleman who did so much for me in the way of knowledge, even though he did but little for me in the way of results.

After leaving Philadelphia, I visited Pittsburgh, Baltimore, Washington, New York, Boston and other eastern cities, searching for a cure, but did not find it. I was benefited very little. These experiences, however, all possessed a certain value, although I did not know it at the time. They taught me the things which would not work and by a simple process of elimination I later found the things which would.

Finally, however, having become disgusted with my eastern trip, I bought a ticket for home and boarded the train more nearly convinced than ever that I had an incurable case of stammering.

Some time after trying my experiment with the eastern schools, I saw the advertisement of a professor from Chicago saying that he would be at Fort Wayne, Indiana, (which was 40 miles from my home), for a week.

He was there. So was I. But to my sorrow. I paid him twenty dollars for which he taught me a few simple breathing and vocal exercises, most of which I already knew by heart, having been drilled in them time and again. This fellow was like so many others who claimed to cure stammering--he was in the business just because there were stammerers to cure, and not because he knew anything about it. He treated the effects of the trouble and did not attempt to remove the cause. The fact of the matter is, I doubt whether he knew anything about the cause.

Then one Sunday while reading a Cincinnati Sunday newspaper, I ran across an advertisement of a School of Elocution, in which was the statement, "Stammering Positively Cured!" Whenever I saw a sign "Vocal Culture" I became interested, so I clipped the advertisement, corresponded with the school and not many Sundays later, being able to secure excursion rates to Cincinnati, I made the trip and prepared to begin my work.

The cost of the course was only fifty dollars and I thought I would he getting cured mighty cheap if I succeeded. So I gave this school a "whirl" with the idea of going hack home in a short time cured--to the surprise of my family and friends. But I was doomed to disappointment. I took the twenty lessons, but went home stammering as badly as ever. You can imagine how I felt as the Big Four train whistled at the Wabash river just before pulling into the Wabash station, where I was to get off.

Here was another failure that could be checked up against the instructor who knew nothing whatever about the cause of stammering. The whole idea of the course was to cultivate voice and make me an orator. That was very fine and would, no doubt, have done me a great deal of good, but it was of no use to try to cultivate a fine voice until I could use that voice in the normal way. The finest voice in the world is of no use if you stammer, and cannot use it. The school of elocution went the same way as all the rest--it was a total failure so far as curing my stammering was concerned.

By this time, my effort to be cured of stammering had become a habit, just as eating and sleeping are habits. I was determined to be cured. I made up my mind I would never give up. True, I often said to myself, "I may never be cured," but in the same breath I resolved that if I was not, it could never be said that it was because I was a "quitter."

My next experiment was with a man who claimed he could cure my stammering in one hour. Think of it. Here I had been, spending weeks and months trying out just ONE way of cure and here was a man who could do the whole job IN ONE HOUR. Wonderful power he must possess, I thought. Of course, I did not believe he could do it. I COULD not believe it. It was not believable. But nevertheless, in my effort to be cured, I had resolved to leave no stone unturned. I made up my mind that the only way to be sure that I was not missing the successful method was to try them all.

So I put myself under this man's hand. He was a hypnotist. He felt able to restore speech with a hypnotic sleep and the proper hypnotic suggestion while I was in the trance. But like all the fake fol-de-rol with which I had come in contact, he did not even make an impression.

I will say in behalf of this hypnotic stammer doctor, however, that he was following distinguished precedent in attempting to cure stammering by hypnotism. German professors in particular have been especially zealous in following out this line of endeavor and many of them have written volumes on the subject only to end up with the conclusion (in their own minds, at least) that it is a failure. Hypnotism may be said to be a condition where the will of the subject is entirely dormant and his every act and thought controlled by the mind of the hypnotist. I do not know, not having been conscious at the time, but it is not improbable that while in the hypnotic state, I was able to talk without stammering, since my words were directed by the mind of the professor, and not my own mind. But inasmuch as I couldn't have the professor carried around with me through the rest of my lifetime in order to use his mind, the treatment could not benefit me.

I next got in touch with an honest-looking old man with a beard like one of the prophets, who assured me with a great deal of professional dignity, that stammering was a mere trifle for a magnetic healer like himself and that he could cure it entirely in ten treatments. So I planked down the specified amount for ten treatments, and went to him regularly three times a week for almost a month, when he explained to me, again with a plenitude of professionalism, that my case was a very peculiar one and that it would require ten more treatments. But I could not figure out how, if ten treatments had done me no good, ten more would do any better. So I declined to try his methods any further. Once again I said to myself, "Well, this has failed, too--I wonder what next?"

The next happened to be electrical treatments. When I visited the electrical treatment specialist, he explained to me in a very effective manner just how (according to his views) stammering was caused by certain contractions of the muscles of the vocal organs, etc., and told me that his treatment surely was the thing to eliminate this contraction and leave my speech entirely free from stammering. I knew something about my stammering then, but not a great deal--consequently his explanation sounded plausible to me and appealed to me as being very sensible and so I decided to give it a trial. I was glad after it was over that I had received no bad effects--that was ALL the cause I had to be glad, for he had not changed my stammering one iota, nor had he changed my speech in any way to make it easier for me to talk. Thus, had I found another one of the things that will not work and chalked up another failure against my attempts to be cured of stammering.

By this time, the reader may well wonder why I was not discouraged in my efforts to be cured. Well, who will say that I was not? I believe I was--as far as it was possible for me to be discouraged at that time. But despite all my failures, I had made up my mind never to give up until I was cured of stammering. I set myself doggedly to the task of ridding myself of an impediment that I knew would always hold me down and prevent any measure of success. I stayed with this task. I never gave up. I kept this one thing always hi mind. It was a life job with me if necessary-- and I was not a "quitter." So failures and discouragements simply steeled me to more intense endeavors to be cured. And while these endeavors cost my parents many hundreds of dollars and cost me many years of time, still, I feel today that they were worth while--not worth while enough to go through again, or worth while enough to recommend to any one else--but at least not a total loss to me.

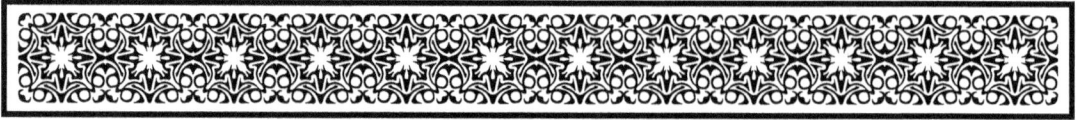

CHAPTER VI
I REFUSE TO BE DISCOURAGED

After I had tried the electric treatment and found it wanting, I heard of a clairvoyant who could, by looking at a person, tell his name, age, occupation, place of residence, etc., and could cure all diseases and afflictions including stammering. So I thought I would give him a trial. He claimed to work through a "greater power"--whatever that was--and so I paid him his fee to see the "greater power" work--and to be cured of stammering, as per promise. But there was nothing doing in the line of a cure--all I got in trying to be cured, was another chapter added to my book of experience.

Following this experience, I tried an osteopath, whose methods, however good they might have been, affected merely the physical organs and could not hope to reach the real cause of my trouble. I do not doubt that this man was entirely sincere in explaining his own science to me in a way that led me to build up hopes of relief from that method. He simply did not understand stammering and its causes and was therefore not prepared to treat it.

I was told of another doctor who claimed to be able to cure stammering. When I called to see him, he had me wait in his reception room for nearly two hours, for the purpose, I presume, of giving me the impression that he was a very busy man. Then he called me into his private consultation room, where he apparently had all of the modern and up-to-date surgical instruments. He put me through a thorough examination, after which he said that the only thing to cure me was a surgical operation to have my tonsils removed. I was not willing to consent to the use of the knife, so therefore the operation was never performed.

Since that time, however, the practice of operating on children especially for the removal of adenoids and tonsils has become very popular and quite frequently this is the remedy prescribed for various and sundry ailments of childhood. In no case must a parent expect to eradicate stuttering or stammering by the removal of the tonsils. The operation, beneficial as it may be in other ways, does not prevent the child from stammering--for the operation does not remove the cause of the stammering--that cause is mental, not physical.

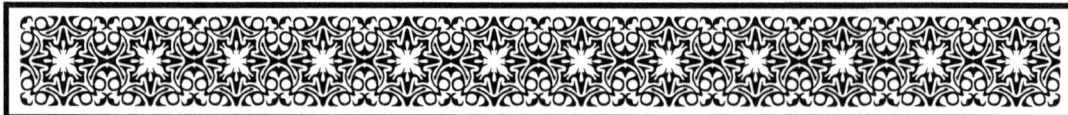

CHAPTER VII
THE BENEFIT OF MANY FAILURES

I had now tried upwards of fifteen different methods for the cure of my stammering. I had tried the physician; the surgeon; the elocution teacher; the hypnotic specialist; the osteopath; a clairvoyant; a mail-order scheme; the world's greatest speech specialist--so-called, and several other things. My parents had spent hundreds of dollars of money trying to have me cured. They had spared no effort, stopped at no cost. And yet I now stammered worse than I had ever stammered before. Everything I had tried had been a worthless failure. Nothing had been of the least permanent good to me. My money was gone, months of time had been wasted and I now began to wonder if I had not been very foolish indeed, in going to first one man and then another, trying to be cured. "Wouldn't it have been better," I asked, "if I had resigned myself to a life as a stammerer and let it go at that?"

My father before me stammered. So did my grandfather and no less than fourteen of my blood relations. My affliction was inherited and therefore supposedly incurable. At least so I was told by honest physicians and other scientific observers who believed what they said and who had no desire to make any personal gain by trafficking in my infirmity. These men told me frankly that their skill and knowledge held out no hope for me and advised me from the very beginning to save my money and avoid the pitfalls of the many who would profess to be able to cure me.

But I had disregarded this honest advice, sincerely given, had spent my money and my time--and what had I gotten? Would I not have been better off if I had listened to the advice and stayed at home? Everything seemed to answer "Yes," but down in my heart I felt that things were better as they were. Certainly some good must come of all this effort--surely it could not all be wasted.

"But yet," I argued with myself, "what good can come of it?" Stammering was fast ruining my life. It had already taken the joy out of my childhood and had made school a task almost too heavy to be undertaken. It had marked my youth with a somber melancholy, and now that youth was slipping away from me with no hope that the future held anything better for me than the past. Something had to be done. I was overpowered by that thought--something had to be done. It had to be done at once. I had come to the turning point in my life. Like Hamlet, I found myself repeating over and over again,

"To be or not to be,   That is the question."

Was I discouraged? No, I will not admit that I was discouraged, but I was pretty nearly resigned to a life without fluent speech, nearly convinced that future efforts to find a cure for stammering would be fruitless and bring no better results.

It was about this time that I stepped into the office of my cousin, then a successful lawyer and district attorney of his city, later the first vice-president of one of the great American railroads with headquarters in New York, and now retired. He was one of those men in whose vocabulary there is no such word as "fail." After I had talked with him for quite a while, he looked at me, and with his kindly, almost fatherly smile asked, "Why don't you cure yourself?"

"Cure myself?" I queried. "How do you expect me, a young man with no scientific training, to cure myself, when the learned doctors, surgeons and scientists of the country hare given me up as incurable?"

"That doesn't make any difference," he replied, "'while there is life, there is hope' and it's a sure thing that nobody ever accomplished anything worth while by accepting the failures of others as proof that the thing couldn't be done. Whitney would never have invented the cotton gin if he had accepted the failures of others as final. Columbus picked out a road to America and assured the skeptics that there was no danger of his sailing 'over the edge.' Of course, it had never been done before, but then Columbus went ahead and did it himself. He didn't take somebody else's failure as an indication of what he could do. If he had, a couple of hundred years later, somebody else would have discovered it and put Columbus in the class with the rest of the weak-kneed who said it couldn't BE done, just because IT NEVER HAD BEEN DONE.

"The progress of this country, Ben," continued my cousin, "is founded on the determination of men who refuse to accept the failures of others as proof that things can't be done at all. Now you've got a mighty good start. You've found out all about these other methods--you know that they have failed--and in a lot of cases, you know WHY they have failed. Now, why don't you begin where they have left off and find out how to succeed?"

The thought struck me like a bolt from a clear sky: "BEGIN WHERE THE OTHERS LEAVE OFF AND FIND OUT HOW TO SUCCEED!" I kept saying it over and over to myself, "Begin where the others leave off-- begin where the others leave off!"

This thought put high hope in my heart. It seemed to ring like a call from afar. "Begin where the others leave off and find out how to succeed." I kept thinking about that all the way home. I thought of it at the table that evening. I said nothing. I went to bed--but I didn't go to sleep, for singing through my brain was that sentence, "Begin where the others leave off and find out how to succeed!"

Right then and there I made the resolve that resulted in my curing myself. "I WILL do it," I said, "I will begin where the others leave off--and I WILL SUCCEED!!" Then and there I determined to master the principles of speech, to chart the methods that had been used by others, to find their defects, to locate the cause of stammering, to find out how to remove that cause and remove it from myself, so that I, like the others whom I so envied, could talk freely and fluently.

That resolution--that determination which first fired me that evening never left me. It marked the turning point in my whole life. I was no longer dependent upon others, no longer looking to physicians or elocution teachers or hypnotists to cure me of stammering. I was looking to myself. If I was to be cured, then I must be the one to do it. This responsibility sobered me. It intensified my determination. It emphasized in my own mind the need for persistent effort, for a constant striving toward this one thing. And absorbed with this idea, living and working toward this one end, I began my work.

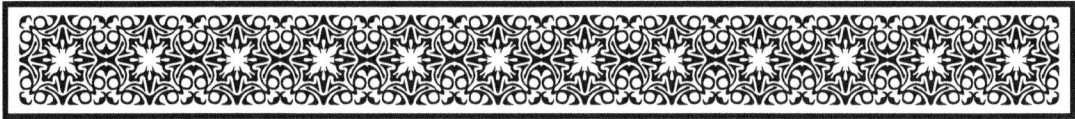

CHAPTER VIII
BEGINNING WHERE OTHERS HAD LEFT OFF

From the moment that my resolution took shape, my plans were all laid with one thing in mind--to cure myself of stammering. I determined, first of all, to master the principles of speech. I remembered very well, indeed, the admonition of Prof. J. J. Mills, President of Earlham College, on the day I left the institution. "You have been a hard-working student," he said, "but your success will never be complete until you learn to talk as others talk. Cure your stammering at any cost." That was the thing I had determined to do. And having determined upon that course, I resolved to let nothing swerve me from it.

I began the study of anatomy. I studied the lungs, the throat, the brain--nothing escaped me. I pursued my studies with the avidity of the medical student wrapped up in his work. I read all the books that had been published on the subject of stammering. I sought eagerly for translations of foreign books on the subject. I lived in the libraries. I studied late at night and arose early in the morning, that I might be at my work again. It absorbed me. I thought of the subject by day and dreamed of it by night. It was never out of my mind. I was living it, breathing it, eating it. I had not thought myself capable of such concentration as I was putting in on the pursuit of the truth as regards stammering and its cure.

With the knowledge that I had gained from celebrated physicians, specialists and institutions throughout this country and Europe, I extended my experiments and investigation. I had an excellent subject on which to experiment--myself. Progress was slow at first--so slow, in fact, that I did not realize until later that it was progress at all. Nothing but my past misery, backed up by my present determination to be free from the impediment that hampered me at every turn, could have kept me from giving up. But at last, after years of effort, after long nights of study and days of research, I was rewarded by success--I found and perfected a method of control of the articulatory organs as well as of the brain centers controlling the organs of speech. I had learned the cause of stammering and stuttering.

All of the mystery with which the subject had been surrounded by so-called specialists, fell away. In all its clearness, I saw the truth. I saw how the others, who had failed in my case, had failed because of ignorance. I saw that they had been treating effects, not causes. I saw exactly WHY their methods had not succeeded and could never succeed.

In truth I had BEGUN WHERE THE OTHERS LEFT OFF AND WON SUCCESS. The reader can imagine what this meant to me. It meant that at last I could speak--clearly, distinctly, freely, and fluently, without those facial contortions that had made me an object of ridicule wherever I went. It meant that I could take my place in life, a man among men; that I could look the whole world in the face; that I could live and enjoy life as other normal persons lived and enjoyed it.

At first my friends could not believe that my cure was permanent. Even my mother doubted the evidence of her own ears. But I knew the trouble would not come back, for the old fear was gone, the nervousness soon passed away, and a new feeling of confidence and self-reliance took hold of me, with the result that in a few weeks I was a changed man. People who had formerly avoided me because of my infirmity began to greet me with new interest. Gradually the old affliction was forgotten by those with whom I came into daily contact and by many I was thought of as a man who had never stammered. Even today, those who knew me when I stammered so badly I could hardly talk, are hardly able to believe that I am the same person who used to be known as "BEN BOGUE'S BOY WHO STUTTERS."

For today I can talk as freely and fluently as anybody. I do not hesitate in the least. For years, I have not even known what it is to grope mentally for a word. I speak in public as well as in private conversation. I have no difficulty in talking over the telephone and in fact do not know the difference. In my work, I lecture to students and am invited to address scientific bodies, societies and educational gatherings, all of which I can accomplish without the slightest difficulty.

Today, I can say with Terence, "I am a man and nothing that is human is alien to me." And I can go a step further and say to those who are afflicted as I was afflicted: "I have been a stammerer. I know your troubles, your sorrows, your discouragements. I understand with an understanding born of a costly experience."

Man or woman, boy or girl, wherever you are, my heart goes out to you. Whatever your station in life, rich or poor, educated or unlettered, discouraged and hopeless, or determined and resolute, I send you a message of hope, a message which, in the words of Dr. Russell R. Conwell, "has been affirmed and reaffirmed in the thousands of lives I have been privileged to watch. And the message is this: Neither heredity nor environment nor any obstacles superimposed by man can keep you from marching straight through to a cure, provided you are guided by a firm driving determination and have normal health and intelligence." To that end I commend to you the succeeding pages of this volume, where you will find in plain and simple language the things which I have spent more than thirty years in learning. May these pages open for you the door to freedom of speech--as they have opened it for hundreds before you.

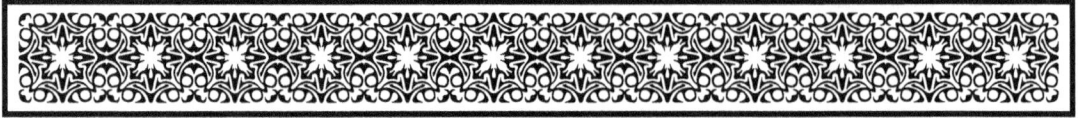

PART II
STAMMERING AND STUTTERING
The Causes, Peculiarities, Tendencies and Effects

CHAPTER I
SPEECH DISORDERS DEFINED

In the diagnosis of speech disorders, there are almost as many different forms of defective utterance as there are cases, all of which forms, however, divide themselves into a few basic types. These various disorders might be broadly classified into three classes:

(1)--Those resulting from carelessness in learning to speak;
(2)--Those which are of distinct mental form; and
(3)--Those caused by a physical deformity in the organs of
speech themselves.

Regardless of under which of these three heads a speech disorder may come, it is commonly spoken of by the laymen as a "speech impediment" or "a stoppage in speech" notwithstanding the fact that the characteristics of the various disorders are quite dissimilar. In certain of the disorders,

(a)--There is an inability to release a word; in others,
(b)--A tendency to repeat a syllable several times before
the following syllable can be uttered; in others,

(c)--The tendency to substitute an incorrect sound for the
   correct one; while in others,

(d)--The utterance is defective merely in the imperfect
   enunciation of sounds and syllables due to some organic
   defect, or to carelessness in learning to speak.

While this volume has but little to do with speech disorders other than stammering and stuttering, the characteristics of the more common forms of speech impediment--lisping, cluttering and hesitation, as well as stuttering and stammering--will be discussed in this first chapter, in order that the reader may be able, in a general way at least, to differentiate between the various disorders.

LISPING

This is a very common form of speech disorder and one which manifests itself early in the life of the child. Lisping may be divided into three forms:

(1)--Negligent Lisping
(2)--Neurotic Lisping
(3)--Organic Lisping

NEGLIGENT LISPING: This is a form of defective enunciation caused in most cases by parental neglect or the carelessness of the child himself in the pronunciation of words during the first few months of talking. This defective pronunciation in Negligent Lisping is caused either by a FAILURE or an INABILITY to observe others who speak correctly. We learn to speak by imitation, and failing to observe the correct method of speaking in others, we naturally fail to speak correctly ourselves. In Negligent Lisping, this inability properly to imitate correct speech processes, results in the substitution of an incorrect sound for the correct one with consequent faulty formation of words.

ORGANIC LISPING: This results from an organic or physical defect in the vocal organs, such as hare-lip, feeble lip, malformation of the tongue, defective teeth, overshot or undershot jaw, high palatal arch, cleft palate, defective palate, relaxed palate following an operation for adenoids, obstructed nasal passages or defective hearing.

NEUROTIC LISPING: This is a form of speech marked by short, rapid muscular contractions instead of the smooth and easy action used in producing normal sounds. Neurotic Lisping is often found to be combined with stammering or stuttering, which is quite logical, since it is similar, both as to CAUSE and as to the presence of a MENTAL DISTURBANCE. In Neurotic Lisping, the muscular movements are less spasmodic than in cases of stuttering, partaking more of the cramped sticking movement, common in stammering.

STUTTERING

Stuttering may be generally defined as the repetition--rapid in some cases, slow in others--of a word or a syllable, before the following word or syllable can be uttered. Stuttering may take several forms, any one of which will fall into one of four phases:

(1)--Simple Phase
(2)--Advanced Phase
(3)--Mental Phase
(4)--Compound Phase

Simple stuttering can be said to be a purely physical form of the difficulty. The Advanced Phase marks the stage of further progress where the trouble passes from the purely physical state into a condition that may be known as Mental-Physical. The distinctly Mental Phase is marked by symptoms indicating a mental cause for the trouble, the disorder usually having passed into this form from the simple or advanced stages of the malady. Stuttering may be combined with stammering in which case the condition represents the Compound Phase of the trouble.

CHOREATIC STUTTERING: This originates in an attack of Acute Chorea or St. Vitus Dance, which leaves the sufferer in a condition where involuntary and spasmodic muscular contractions, especially of the face, have become an established habit. This breaks up the speech in a manner somewhat similar to ordinary stuttering. Also known as "Tic Speech."

SPASTIC SPEECH: This is often the result of infantile cerebral palsy, the characteristic symptom of the trouble being intense over-exertion, continued throughout a sentence, the syllables being equal in length and very laboriously enunciated. In spastic speech, there is present a noticeable hyper-tonicity of the nerve fibers actuating the muscles used in speaking as well as marked contractions of the facial muscles.

UNCONSCIOUS STUTTERING: This is a misnomer because there can be no such thing as unconscious stuttering. It appears that the person afflicted is not conscious of his difficulty for he insists that he does not s-s-s-tut-tut-tut-ter. Unconscious Stuttering is but a name for the disorder of a stutterer who is too stubborn to admit his own difficulty.

THOUGHT STUTTERING: This is an advanced form of stuttering which is also known as Aphasia and which is caused by the inability of the sufferer to recall the mental images necessary to the formation of a word. Stuttering in its simpler forms is usually connected with the period of childhood, while aphasia is often connected with old age or injury. The aphasic person is excessively nervous as is the stutterer; he undergoes the same anxiety to get his words out and the same fear of being ridiculous. In aphasia there is, however, no excessive muscular tension or cramp of the speech muscles. In these cases, the stutterer will sometimes repeat the first syllable ten or fifteen times with pauses between, being for a time unable to recall what the second syllable is. It is, in other words, a habitual, but nevertheless temporary, inability to recall to mind the mental images necessary to produce the word or syllable desired to be spoken. This condition is more commonly known as Thought Lapse or the inability to think of what you desire to say.

One investigator shows that the diagnosis of "insanity" with later commitment to an asylum occurred in the case of a bad stutterer. When excited he would go through the most extreme contortions and the wildest gesticulations in a vain attempt to finally get all of the word out, finally pacing up and down the room like one truly insane. This tendency to believe that the stutterer is insane because of the convulsive or spasmodic effort accompanying his efforts to speak, is a mistaken one, although there can be little doubt of the tendency of this condition finally to lead to insanity if not checked.

HESITATION

Hesitation is marked by a silent, choking effort, often accompanied by a fruitless opening and closing of the mouth. Hesitation is a stage through which the sufferer usually passes before he reaches the condition known as Elementary Stammering.

STAMMERING

Stammering is a condition in which the person afflicted is unable to begin a word or a sentence no matter how much effort may be directed toward the attempt to speak, or how well they may know what they wish to say. In stammering, there is the "sticking" as the stammerer terms it, or the inability to express a sound. The difference between stammering and stuttering lies in the fact that in stuttering, the disorder manifests itself in loose and hurried (or in some cases, slow) repetitions of sounds, syllables or words, while in the case of stammering, the manifestation takes the form of an inability to express a sound, or to begin a word or a sentence.

ELEMENTARY STAMMERING: This is the simplest form of this disorder. Here, the convulsive effort is not especially noticeable and the marked results of long-continued stammering are not apparent. Most cases pass quickly from the elementary stage unless checked in their incipiency.

SPASMODIC STAMMERING: This marks the stage of the disorder where the effort to speak brings about marked muscular contractions and pronounced spasmodic efforts, resulting in all sorts of facial contortions, grimaces and uncontrolled jerkings of the head, body and limbs.

THOUGHT STAMMERING: This, like Thought-Stuttering, is a form of Aphasia and manifests itself in the inability of the stammerer to think of what he wishes to say. In other words, the thought- stammerer, like the thought-stutterer, is unable

to recall the mental images necessary to the production of a certain word or sound--
and is, therefore, unable to produce sounds correctly. The manifestations described
under Thought Stuttering are present in Thought Stammering also.

COMBINED STAMMERING AND STUTTERING: This is a compound form
of difficulty in which the sufferer finds himself at times not only unable to utter a
sound or begin a word or a sentence but also is found to repeat a sound or syllable
several times before the following syllable can be uttered. Any case of stuttering or
stammering in the Simple or Elementary Stages may pass into Combined Stammering and Stuttering without warning or without the knowledge, even, of the stammerer or stutterer.

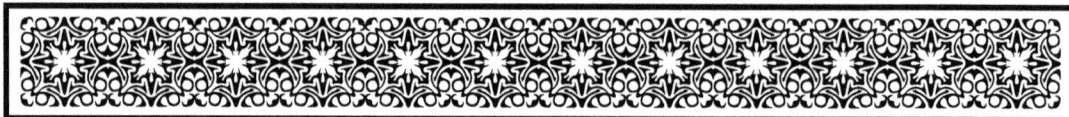

CHAPTER II
THE CAUSES OF STUTTERING AND STAMMERING

One of the first questions asked by the stutterer or stammerer is, "What is the cause of my trouble?" In asking this question, the stammerer is getting at the very essence of the successful method of treatment of his malady, for there is no method of curing stuttering, stammering and kindred defects of speech that can bring real and permanent relief from the affliction unless it attacks the cause of the trouble and removes that cause.

Inasmuch as this book has to do almost entirely with the two defective forms of utterance known as stuttering and stammering, we will at this time drop all reference to the other forms of speech impediments and from this time forth refer only to stuttering and stammering.

These forms of defective speech are manifested by the inability to express words in the normal, natural manner--freely and fluently. In other words, there is a marked departure from the normal in the methods used by the stammerer in the production of speech. It is necessary, therefore, before taking up the discussion of the causes of stuttering and stammering, to determine the method by which voice is produced in the normal individual, so that we can compare this normal production of speech with the faulty method adopted by the stutterer or stammerer and learn where the fault is and what is the cause of it.

Let us now proceed to do this: In other words, let us ask the question: "How is speech produced in the normal person not afflicted with defective utterance?"

Voice is produced by the vocal organs much in the same manner as sounds are produced on a saxophone or clarinet, by forcing a current of air through an aperture over which is a reed which vibrates with the sounds. The low tones produced by the saxophone or clarinet result from the enlargement of the aperture, while the higher tones are produced by contracting the opening. Variations of pitch in the human voice are also effected by elongation and contraction of the vocal cords with comparative slackness or tension, as in the violin.

It would be of no value, and, in fact, would only serve to confuse the layman, to know the duties or functions of the various organs or parts entering into the production of speech. Suffice it to say that in the "manufacture" of words, there are concerned the glottis, the larynx, thorax, diaphragm, lungs, soft palate, tongue, teeth and lips. In the production of the sounds and the combination of sounds that we call words, each of these organs of speech has its own particular duty to perform and the failure of any one of these organs properly to perform that duty may result in defective utterance of some form.

BRAIN CONTROL: It must be borne in mind that for any one or all of the organs of speech to become operative or to manifest any action, they must be innervated or activated by impulses originating in the brain.

For instance, if it is necessary that the glottis be contracted to a point which we will call "half-open" for the production of a certain sound, the brain must first send a message to that organ before the necessary movement can take place. In saying the word "you," for instance, it would be necessary for the tongue to press tip against the base of the lower row of front teeth. But before the tongue can assume that position, it is necessary that the brain send to the tongue a message directing what is to be done.

When the number of different organs involved in the production of the simplest word of one syllable is considered (such as the word "you" just mentioned), and when it is further considered that separate brain messages must be sent to each of the organs, muscles or parts concerned in the production of that word, then it will be understood that the process of speaking is a most complicated one, involving not only numerous physical organs but also intricate mental processes.

When all of the organs concerned in the production of speech are working properly and when the brain sends prompt and correct brain impulses to them, the result is perfect speech, the free, fluent and easy conversation of the good talker. But when any or all of these organs fail to function properly, due to inco-ordination, the result is discord--and defective utterance.

CAUSE OF DEFECTIVE UTTERANCE: Now, let us consider the cause of defective utterance. What is it that causes the organ, muscle or parts to fail properly to function? The first and most obvious conclusion would be that there was some inherent defect in the organ, muscle or part which failed to function. But experience has proved that this is usually not the case. An examination of two thousand cases of defective utterance, including many others besides stuttering and stammering, revealed three-tenths of one per cent. with an organic defect--that is, a defect in the organs themselves. In other words, only three persons out of every thousand afflicted with defective utterance were found to have any physical shortcoming that was responsible for the affliction.

Take any of these two thousand cases--say those that stammered, for instance. What was the cause of their difficulty, if it did not lie in the organs used in the production of speech? This is the question that long puzzled investigators in the field of speech defects. Like Darwin, they said: "It must be this, for if it is not this, then what is it?" If stuttering and stammering are not caused by actual physical defects in the organs themselves, what then can be the cause?

DUE TO A LACK OF CO-ORDINATION: Cases of stammering and stuttering where no organic defect is present are due to a lack of co- ordination between the brain and the muscles of speech. In other words, the harmony between the brain and the speech organs which normally result in smooth working and perfect speech has been interrupted. The brain impulses are no longer properly transmitted to and executed by the muscles of speech.

This failure to transmit properly brain messages or this lack of co-ordination may take one of two forms: it may result in an UNDER-innervation of the organs of speech, which results in loose, uncontrolled repetitions of a word, sound or syllable, or it may take the form of an overinnervation of the vocal organ with the result that it is so intensely contracted as to be entirely closed, causing the "sticking" or inability to pronounce even a sound, so common to the stammerer.

Suppose that you try to say the word "tray." Do not articulate the sounds. Merely make the initial effort to say it. What happens? Simply this: The tip of the tongue comes in contact with the upper front teeth at their base and as you progress in your attempt to say "t," the tongue flattens itself against the roof of the mouth, moving from the tip of the tongue toward its base. If you are a stammerer, you will probably find in endeavoring to say this word, that your vocal organs fail to respond quickly and correctly to the set of brain messages which should result in the proper enunciation of the word "tray." Your tongue clings to the roof of your mouth, your mouth remains open, you suffer a rush of blood to the face, due to your powerful and unsuccessful effort to articulate, and the word refuses to be spoken.

Now, in order to dissociate "lack of co-ordination," from stammering and to get an idea of its real nature, let us imagine an experiment which can be conducted by any one, whether they stammer or not.

You see on the table before you a pencil. You want to write and consequently you want to pick up the pencil. Therefore, your brain sends a message to your thumb and forefinger, saying, "Pick up the pencil." Your brain does not, of course, express that command in words, but sends a brain impulse based upon the kinaesthetic or motor image of the muscular action necessary to accomplish that act. But for our purpose in this experiment, we can assume that the brain sends the message in terms which, if interpreted in words, would be "pick up the pencil." Suppose that when that brain message reaches your thumb and forefinger, instead of reaching for the pencil, they immediately close and clap or stick, refusing to act. Your hand is unable to pick up the pencil. That, then, is similar to stammering. The hand is doing practically what the vocal organs do when the stammerer attempts to speak and fails. But, on the other hand, if, when the message was received by your thumb and finger, it made short, successive attempts to pick up the pencil, but failed to accomplish it, then you could compare that failure to the uncontrolled repetitions of stuttering. This inability to control the action of the thumb and forefinger would be the result of a lack of co-ordination between the brain and the muscles of the hand, while stuttering or stammering is the result of a lack of co-ordination between the brain and the muscles of speech.

WHAT CAUSES LACK OF CO-ORDINATION: But even after it is known that stuttering and stammering are caused by a lack of co-ordination between the brain and the organs of speech, still, the mind of scientific and inquiring trend must ask, "What causes the lack of co-ordination?" And that question is quite in order. It is plain that the lack of co-ordination does not exist without a cause. What, then, is this cause?

An inquiry into the cause of the inco-ordination between brain and speech-organs leads us to an examination of the original or basic causes of stammering.

These original or basic causes in their various ramifications are almost as numerous as the cases of speech disorders themselves, but they fall into a comparatively few well-defined classes.

These original causes in many cases do not appear to have been the direct and immediate cause of the trouble, but rather a predisposing cause or a cause which brought about a condition that later developed into stuttering or stammering.

Let us set down a list of the more common of these causes, not with the expectation of having the list complete but rather of giving facts about the representative or more common Basic Predisposing Causes of Stuttering and Stammering.

A little more than 96 per cent. of the causes of stammering which the author has examined can be traced back to one of the five causes shown below:

    1--Mimicry or Imitation
    2--Fright or severe nerve shock
    3--Fall or injury of some sort
    4--Heredity
    5--Disease

Let us take up these familiar causes of stuttering or stammering in the order in which we have set them down and learn something more of them.

The first and one of the most common causes is Mimicry, or, as it is probably more often called, Imitation. Mimicry or Imitation is almost wholly confined to children. After reaching the age of discretion, the adult is usually of sufficient intelligence to refrain from mimicking or imitating a person who stutters or stammers.

The average small boy, however, (or girl, for that matter) seems to find delight in mocking and imitating a playmate who stutters or stammers, and so keen is this delight that he persists in this practice day after day until (as its own punishment) the practice of mockery or mimicry brings upon the boy himself the affliction in which he found his fun.

It may be noted, however, that Imitation is not always conscious, but often unconscious. The small child begins to imitate the stuttering companion without knowing that he engages in imitation. This practice, notwithstanding the fact that it is unconscious, soon develops into stuttering, without any cause being assignable by the parent until investigation develops that unconscious and even unnoticed imitation is the basic cause of the defective utterance.

It has been definitely determined that stuttering may be communicable through contagious impressions, especially among children of tender age whose minds are subject to the slightest impressions.

For this reason, it is not advisable for parents to allow children to play with others who stutter or stammer, nor is it charitable to allow a child who stutters or stammers to play with other children who are not so afflicted.

So far-reaching are the effects of Imitation or Mimicry that in certain cases, children have been known to contract stuttering from associating with a deaf-mute whose expressions were made chiefly in the form of grunts and inarticulate sounds.

FRIGHT OR SEVERE NERVE SHOCK: Another common cause of stammering is fright or nervous shock, which may have been brought about in countless ways. One boy who came to me some time ago stated that he had swallowed a nail when about six years of age and that this was the cause of his stammering. The logical conclusion in a case like this would be that the nail had injured the vocal organs, but an examination proved that there was no organic defect and that the stammering was caused, not by injury directly to the vocal organs but by the nervous shock occasioned by swallowing the nail.

Another case was that of a stammerer who reported that he had been given carbolic acid, by mistake, when a child and that he had stammered ever since. This, like the case of the boy who swallowed the nail, might be expected to prove a case of absolute physical injury or impairment of the vocal chords, but once again, it was clear that such was not the case and that the stammering was brought about solely from the nervous shock which came as a result of taking carbolic acid.

There is still another case of a boy who felt that he was continually being followed. This was of course merely a hallucination, but the fright that this boy's state of mind brought on soon caused him to stutter and stammer in a very pronounced manner.

Fright is a prolific cause of stuttering in small children and may be traced in a great many cases to parents or nurses who persist in telling children stories of a frightful nature, or who, as a means of discipline, scare them by locking them up in the cellar, the closet or the garret. To these scare-tales told to children should be added the misguided practice of telling children that "the bogey-man will get you" or "the policeman is after you" or some such tale to enforce parental commands. An instance is recalled of a woman who created out of a morbid imagination a phantom of terrible mien, who abode in the garret and was constantly lying in wait for the small children of the household with the professed intention of "eating them alive."

Such disciplinary methods of parents savor much of the Inquisition and the Dark Ages and should, for the good of the children and the future generation they represent, be totally abolished. While these methods do not, in every case, result in stuttering or stammering, they make the child of a nervous disposition and lay him liable in later years to the afflictions which accompany nervous disorders. In some cases "tickling" a child has caused stammering or stuttering. Care should be exercised here as well, for prolonged tickling brings about intense muscular contraction especially of the diaphragmatic muscles, which contraction is accompanied by an agitated mental condition as well as extreme nervousness, all of which approaches very closely to the combination of abnormal conditions which are found to be present in stammering or stuttering.

FALL OR INJURY AS A CAUSE: Step into any gathering of average American parents for a half-hour and if the subject of the children should come up, you are sure to hear one or more dramatic recitals of the falls and injuries suffered by the junior members of the household, from the first time that Johnny fell out of bed and frightened his mother nearly to death, to the day that he was in an automobile crash at the age of 23. And these tales are always closed with the profound bit of confided information that these falls are of no consequence--"nothing ever comes of them."

While in a great measure this is true, there are many falls and injuries suffered in childhood which are responsible for the ills of later life, although it is seldom indeed that they are blamed for the results which they bring about.

Injuries and falls are a frequent cause of stuttering and stammering. Usually, however, an injury results in stuttering or stammering, not because of any change in the physical structure brought about by the injury but rather by the nervous shock attending it. In other words, cases of stammering and stuttering caused apparently by injury might, if desired, be traced still further back, showing as the initial cause an injury but as a direct cause the fright or nervous shock resulting from that injury.

A good example of this is found in a case of a young man who came to me some years ago. He said: "When I was about five years old, my brother and I were playing in the cellar and I wanted to jump off the top step. When I jumped, I hit my head on the cross-piece and it knocked me back on the steps and I slid down on my back, and ever since, for ten years, I have stammered."

Here is a case where the blow on the head, or the succession of blows on the spinal column as the boy slid down the stairs, might have been the cause of the trouble. More probably, it was the combined injury, undoubtedly resulting in a severe nervous shock from which the boy probably did not recover for many days.

Another man said, in describing his case during an examination: "At the age of 16, I was hit on the head with a ball. I lost my memory for one week and when I regained it, I was a stammerer." This is a plain case of injury resulting in immediate stammering.

Still another case is that of a boy who, at the age of three, was shot in the neck by a rifle, the bullet coming out of his chin, which resulted in his becoming an immediate stammerer. Here, as in the case of the boy who swallowed the nail, it might be expected that the cause was a defect in the organs of speech, but I found stammering was brought on by the nervous shock.

From these few cases of actual occurrences, it will be seen that practically all cases of stammering caused by injury can be traced to the NERVOUS SHOCK brought about by the injury.

HEREDITY AS A CAUSE: There is little that need be said on the subject of heredity as a cause of stuttering and stammering, save that heredity is a common cause and that children of stuttering or stammering parents usually stammer. In this, as in the case of any malady hereditarily transmitted, it is difficult to say whether the trouble is caused by inheritance or by constant and intimate association of the child with his parents during the period of early speech development.

THE RESULT OF DISEASE: Many cases of both stammering and stuttering may be traced back to disease as the basic or predisposing cause. Acute Chorea (St. Vitus Dance) is frequently the cause of stuttering of a type known as Choreatic Stuttering or "Tic Speech." Infantile Cerebral Palsy sometimes brings about a condition known as "Spastic Speech," while whooping cough, scarlet fever, measles, meningitis, infantile paralysis, scrofula and rickets are sometimes responsible for the disorder.

Disease may cause stuttering or stammering as an immediate after effect or the speech trouble may not show up for considerable time, depending altogether upon the individual. But regardless of the length of time elasping between the disease which predisposes the individual to the speech disorder and the time of the first evidence of its presence, diagnosis reveals but an insignificant percentage of organic defects in these cases resulting from disease, indicating that even here the predominant causative factor is a mental one.

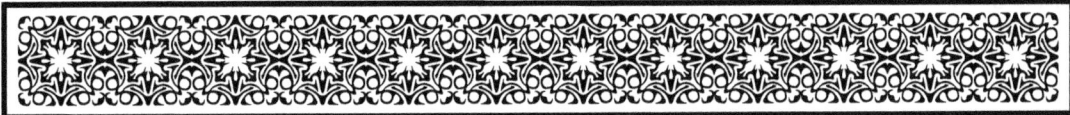

CHAPTER III
THE PECULIARITIES OF STUTTERING AND STAMMERING

Each individual case of stuttering or stammering has its own peculiarities, already more or less developed--arising from structural differences (but not necessarily defects) in the organs of speech, as well as differences in temperament, health and nervousness; or peculiarities arising from habit--which is the result of previous training or neglect, as the case may be.

SING WITHOUT DIFFICULTY: Almost without exception, the stutterer or stammerer can sing without any difficulty, can talk to animals without stuttering or stammering, can talk when alone and in some cases can talk perfectly in a whisper. Some stammerers have less difficulty in talking to strangers than in talking to friends or relatives while in other cases, the condition is exactly reversed. A stutterer or stammerer almost always experiences difficulty in speaking over the telephone. One experimenter has shown, however, that a stammerer can talk perfectly over the telephone so long as the receiver hook is depressed and there is no connection with another person at the other end of the line. This experimenter shows that immediately the receiver hook is released and a connection is established, the halting, stumbling utterance begins.

These peculiarities of stuttering and stammering for many years puzzled investigators and were, in fact, finally responsible for arriving at the true cause of stammering.

Almost every stammerer seeks for an explanation of these peculiar manifestations. Why is it, for instance, that a stammerer can sing without difficulty, although he cannot talk? This is one of the best evidences that could be produced to show that stammering is the result of a lack of mental control. The stammerer who can sing without difficulty has no organic or inherent defect in the vocal organs, that is sure. If the stammerer can sing, and if this proves that he has no organic defect, then it follows logically that the cause of his trouble is mental and not physical.

TALK WHEN ALONE: The fact that a stammerer can talk without hesitation when alone and that he can talk to animals may be explained by a very simple illustration--any stammerer can try this experiment on one of his friends who does not stammer. He can prove that the reflex, or what might be termed subconscious movements of the bodily organs are more nearly normal than the same movements consciously controlled. Take, for instance, the regular beating of the pulse. Let anyone who does not stammer (it makes no difference in trying this experiment whether the person stammers or not, save that we are trying to prove that the condition may be brought about in one who is not a stammerer) feel his own pulse for sixty seconds. Let him be thoroughly conscious of this effort to learn the rapidity of its beating. If a disinterested observer could record the pulse as normally beating and the pulse under the conscious influence of the mind, it would be found that the pulse under the conscious effort is beating either more rapidly or more slowly or that it is not beating as regularly as in the case of unconscious or reflex action.

This same condition may be noticed in another unconscious or reflex action-- breathing. The moment you become conscious of an attempt to breathe regularly, breathing becomes difficult, restricted, irregular, whereas this same action, when unconscious, is thoroughly regular and even.

In the average or normal person who has learned to talk correctly, speaking should be practically an unconscious process. It should not be necessary to make a conscious effort to form words, nor should a normal individual be conscious of the energy necessary to create a word or the muscular movements necessary to its formation and expression.

This will explain why the stutterer or stammerer can talk without difficulty to animals or when alone--there is no self- consciousness--no conscious effort--no thinking of what is being done.

Another of the peculiarities of stammering is that the stammerer in many cases seems to be able to talk perfectly in concert. This has long baffled the investigator in this field, no reason being assignable for this ability to talk in connection with others. The baffling element has been this--that the investigator has assumed that the stammerer talked well in concert, whereas a very careful scientist would have discovered the stammerer to be a fraction of a second or a part of a syllable behind the others.

You have doubtless been in church at some time when you were not entirely familiar with the hymn being sung, yet by lagging a note or two behind the rest, you could sing the song, to all appearances being right along with the others.

When you talk over the long-distance telephone, the voice seems instantly to reach the party at the other end of the line, yet we know that a period of time has had to elapse to allow the voice waves to move along the telephone wire and reach the other end. The elapse of time has been too slight to be noted by the average human mind and the transmission seems instantaneous. This is what happens in the case of the stammerer who seems able to talk in concert--he is merely a syllable or part of a syllable behind the rest, all the while giving the impression nevertheless, that he is talking just as they are.

There are many other individual peculiarities which can be described by almost every stammerer. These different peculiarities are more numerous than the cases of stammering and it would be useless to attempt to discuss them in detail. I will take up only two as being typical of dozens which have come under my observation in twenty-eight years' experience.

One stammerer explains his difficulty as follows: "I find I am unable to talk and do something else at the same time. For instance, I have difficulty in talking while dancing, while at the table or while listening to music. If, for instance, I wish to talk to any one while the Victrola is being played, I unconsciously cut it off." This is a case where the stammerer finds that all of his faculties must be concentrated upon a supreme effort to speak before this becomes possible. In other words, he has not yet learned to control sufficiently the different parts of his body so that they may act independently. This might be termed a lack of independent co-ordination.

In the case of another young man, he found himself unable to control the movements of his muscles. In describing his trouble, he said: "At one time, when I was talking particularly bad, I was out with some other fellows driving our car. I started to talk, found it almost impossible and noticed a sharp twitching of the muscles of face, arms and limbs. Try as I might, I found I could not control these movements and in another minute I had steered the car into the ditch and wrecked it. And now," adds the young man, "although father has a new car, I am never allowed to drive it!"

Here was a case where the spasmodic action of the muscles had gotten so far beyond control as to make the ordinary pursuits of life dangerous to the young man who stammered. These spasmodic movements were always present--he told of one occasion when he was in a barber's chair being shaved. He attempted to say a word or two while the barber was at work upon him, with the result that he lost control of the muscles of face and neck, causing the barber to cut a long gash in his neck.

This was, of course, an abnormal case of spasmodic stammering, evidencing extraordinary muscular contractions of the worst type. In practically every case of stammering some such peculiarity is evident, resulting from the inability of the stammerer's brain to control physical actions.

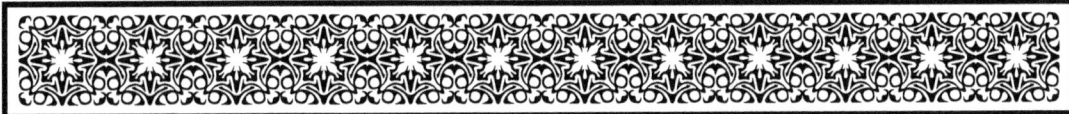

CHAPTER IV
THE INTERMITTENT TENDENCY

Paradoxical as the statement may seem, it is nevertheless true that one of the symptoms of least seeming importance marks one of the most dangerous aspects of both stuttering and stammering.

This is the alternating good-and-bad condition known as the Intermittent Tendency or the tendency of the stutterer or stammerer to show marked improvement at times.

This seeming improvement brings about a feeling of relief, the unreasoning fear of failure seems for the time to have left almost entirely; the mental strain under which the sufferer ordinarily labors seems to be no longer present; there is but little worry about either present condition or future prospects; the nervous condition seems to have very materially improved, self-confidence returns quickly and with it the hope that the trouble is gone forever or is at least rapidly disappearing. With these manifestations of improvement come also a greater ease in concentration, a greater and more facile power-of-will and an ambition that shows signs of rekindling, with worth-while accomplishments in prospect.

Hope now burns high in the breast of the stutterer or stammerer. They go about smiling inwardly if not outwardly, happy as the proud father of a new boy, at peace with the world. The sun shines brighter than it has for months or years. Every one seems much more pleasant and agreeable. Things which the day before seemed totally impossible seem now to come within their range of accomplishment. Such is the feeling of the confirmed stutterer or stammerer during the time of this pseudo-freedom from his speech disorder.

In his own mind, the sufferer is quite sure that his malady has disappeared over-night, like a bad dream and that freedom of speech has been bestowed upon him as a gift from the gods on high.

The higher the hopes of the sufferer and the greater the assurance with which he pursues the activities of his day, the greater is his disappointment and despair when the inevitable relapse overtakes him.

For disappointment and despair are sure to come--just as sure as the sun is to rise in the heavens in the morning. The condition of relief is but temporary, and will soon pass away to be followed by a return of his old trouble in a form more aggravated than ever before.

Fate seems to play with the stammerer's affliction as a cat plays with a mouse, allowing him to be free for a few hours, a few days or a few weeks as the case may be, only to drag the dejected sufferer back to his former condition--or, as is true in many cases, worse than before.

THE RECURRENCE: With the return of the trouble, the bodily and mental reaction are almost too great for the human mechanism to withstand. Hope seems to be a word which has been lost from the life of the stammerer. The fear of failure returns with an overwhelming force mocking the sufferer with the thought of "Oh, how I deceived you!!"; the mental strain is exceedingly great--so great, in fact, that it seems as if the breaking point has almost been reached. The nervous condition is alarming, the sufferer noting in himself an inability to work, to play, to study or even to sit still. An observer would note the stammerer or stutterer in this condition fingering his coat lapels, putting his hands in his pockets and removing them again, biting his finger nails, constantly shifting eyes, head, arms and feet about. If at home, the sufferer in this condition would probably be seen walking about the house, unable to read, to play or listen to music or to follow any of the accustomed activities of his life. If in business or in the shop, he would be noticed making frequent trips to the wash room, to the drinking fountain, to the foreman, picking up and laying down his tools, looking out the window, shifting from one foot to another, all of which symptoms indicate an acute nervous condition, brought about by the return of his trouble.

At this stage, the stammerer's confidence is hopelessly gone, so it seems, and this feeling is accompanied by one of depression which finds an outlet in the expression of the firm belief and conviction on the part of the stutterer or stammerer that the disorder can NEVER be cured, by any method, although just the day before the same sufferer would have insisted that his stuttering or stammering had CURED ITSELF and left of its own accord.

These conditions, both at the time of the so-called improvement and at the time of the recurrence of the trouble, will appear in greater or less degree in the case of every stutterer or stammerer whose trouble is of the intermittent type.

THE DANGERS OF THIS TENDENCY: This period of recurrence is accompanied by almost total loss of the power-of-will, a marked weakening in the ability to concentrate, and if it does not result in insomnia (inability to sleep) puts the mind in such a state as to make sleep of little value in building up the body, replacing worn-out tissue cells and restoring vital energy.

The chief danger, however, resulting from these periods of temporary improvement, is the belief that it instills into the mind of the sufferer and more frequently into the minds of the parents of stuttering or stammering children, that the trouble will cure itself--a fallacy greater than which there is none.

Stuttering and stammering are destructive maladies. They tear down both body and mind but they have not the slightest power to build up. And until a strong mental and physical structure has been built up in place of the weakened structure (which results in stammering and stuttering) a cure is out of the question.

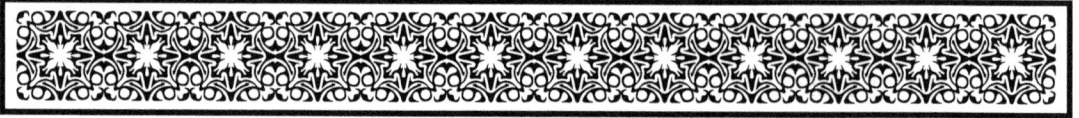

CHAPTER V
THE PROGRESSIVE TENDENCY

The spell of intense recurrence of either stammering or stuttering which follows a period of improvement, often marks the period of transition from one stage of the disorder into the next and more serious stage. This transition, however, may not be a conscious process--that is, the sufferer may not in any way be informed of the fact that he is passing into a more serious stage of his trouble save that after the transition has taken place, he may find himself a chronic or constant stammerer and in a nervous and mental condition much more acute than ever before.

Dr. Alexander Melville Bell (father of Alexander Graham Bell, inventor of the telephone), who, before his death, was a speech expert of unquestioned repute, discovered this condition many years ago and in his work PRINCIPLES OF SPEECH speaks of it as follows (page 234):

"Often the transition from simple to more complicated forms of difficulty is so rapid, that it cannot be traced or anticipated. Perhaps some slight ailment may imperceptibly introduce the higher impediment or some evil example may draw the ill-mastered utterance at onee into the vortex of the difficulty."

This Progressive Tendency, which we shall hereafter call the Progressive Character of the trouble in order to distinguish it from the Intermittent Tendency, is present in more than 98 per cent, of the cases of stammering and stuttering which I have examined and diagnosed.

True, there are many cases, the apparent or manifest tendencies of which do not indicate that the disorder is becoming more serious, but nevertheless this condition is no indication that the trouble is not busily at work tearing out the foundation of mental and bodily perfection.

SUCCESSIVE STAGES: Stuttering may be conveniently divided into four stages, by which its progress may be measured. These may be designated in their order as:

1--Simple Phase
2--Advanced Phase
3--Mental Phase
4--Compound Phase

The progress of the disorder is sure. Take the case of a child eight years of age who has a case of simple stuttering. Permit the child to go without attention for some time and the trouble will have progressed into the Advanced Phase, usually without the knowledge of the child or his parents or without any especially noticeable surface change in his condition.

Stuttering in its first phase--Simple Stuttering--can justly be called a physical and not a mental trouble. In this stage, the disorder should be easily eradicated. The duration of cases of Simple Stuttering is very slight, for the reason that Simple Stuttering soon passes into the Advanced Phase, which is of a physical-mental nature, exhibiting the symptoms of a mental disturbance as well as of a physical difficulty.

From the Advanced Phase stuttering then passes into the Mental Phase, where the mental strain is found to be greatly intensified and the disorder a distinct mental type instead of a physical or physical-mental trouble. When stuttering in this stage is permitted to continue its hold upon the sufferer, the continued strain, worry and fear bring about a condition of extraordinary malignancy, in which the trouble develops into the Chronic Mental Stage. This is a condition bordering upon mental breakdown and even though the complete breakdown never occurs, the one afflicted finds himself a chronic stutterer, without surcease from his trouble. He further finds that he has increasing difficulty in thinking of the things which he wishes to say. He seems to know, but his mind refuses to frame the thought. In other words, he is unable to recall the mental image of the word in mind, and is therefore unable to speak the word. This is a condition known as Aphasia or Thought Lapse and represents a most serious stage of the difficulty, in many cases totally beyond the possibility of relief--a condition in which no stutterer should allow himself to get.

Stammering, being a kindred condition to stuttering, progresses from bad to worse in a manner very similar. The progress of stammering may be classified into successive stages as follows:

    1--Elementary Stage
    2--Spasmodic Stage
    3--Primary Mental Stage
    4--Chronic Mental Stage
    5--Compound Stage

Stammering in the Elementary Stage, like Stuttering, is a Physical Trouble. The Stammerer has often been known to remain in the Elementary Stage only a few days or a few weeks, passing almost immediately into either the Spasmodic or the Primary Mental Stage. Not all stammerers pass into the Spasmodic Stage of the disorder, however, some passing directly into Primary Mental Stage.

The Spasmodic Stage, however, is a form of difficulty somewhat akin to the Advanced Phase of Stuttering, for in this stage the trouble can be said to be of Physical-Mental nature instead of the purely physical disorder found in Elementary Stammering.

Stammering, in the Primary Mental Stage, takes on a distinct Mental form as differentiated from the Mental-Physical form and becomes therefore more difficult to eradicate. If allowed to continue, this form of Stammering (like Stuttering) passes into the Chronic Mental Stage, in which case the Stammerer usually exhibits pronounced signs of Thought Lapse and finds himself a Chronic or Constant Stammerer, often unable to utter a sound-and further at times unable to THINK of what he wishes to say.

The progress of both Stuttering and Stammering from one stage to another is very certain. These speech disorders do not differ materially from other human afflictions in this respect--they do not remain constant. There is an axiom in Nature, that "Nothing is static," which, being interpreted, means, that nothing stands still. And this applies with full force to the stutterer or stammerer. If no steps are taken to remedy the malady, he may be very sure that the disorder is getting worse--not standing still or remaining the same.

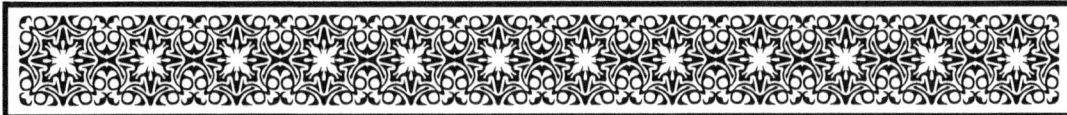

CHAPTER VI
CAN STAMMERING AND STUTTERING
BE OUTGROWN?

Probably the most harmful and oft-repeated bit of advice ever given to a stammerer or stutterer is that which says, "Oh, don't bother about it-- you will soon outgrow the trouble!" It is the most harmful because it is palpably untrue. It is so oft-repeated because the person giving the advice knows nothing whatever about the cause of stammering and just as little about its progress or treatment.

The fact that we hear of no cases of stuttering or stammering which have been outgrown does not seem to alter the popular and totally unfounded belief that stammering and stuttering can be readily outgrown.

If the reader has not read the chapter on the causes of stuttering and stammering and the two preceding chapters on the Intermittent Tendency and the Progressive Character of these speech disorders, then these chapters should be read carefully before going further with this one, because it is essential to know the cause of the trouble before it is possible to answer intelligently the question, "Can Stammering be Outgrown?"

To any one who understands the nature of the difficulty and the progress it is liable to make, the question is almost as absurd as asking whether or not the desire to sleep can be outgrown by staying awake. But aside from its scientific aspect--aside from the absurdity of the question--let us examine the facts as revealed by actual records of cases. Let us dispense with all theory on the subject and take experience gained in a wide range of cases as the correct guide in finding the answer.

FACTS FROM STATISTICS: An examination of the records of several thousand cases of stuttering and stammering of all types and in all stages of development reveals the fact that after passing the age of six, only one-fifth of one per cent, ever outgrow stammering. This means that out of every five hundred people who stammer, only one ever outgrows it. Between the ages of three and six, the indications are more favorable, the records in these cases showing that slightly less than one per cent, outgrow the difficulty. That means that one out of every hundred children affected has a chance, at least, of outgrowing the difficulty between the ages of three and six, and after that time, only one chance in five hundred.

Suppose you were handed a rifle, given five hundred cartridges and told to hit a bull's eye at a hundred yards, 499 times out of 500. Suppose you were told that if you missed once you would have to suffer the rest of your life as a stammerer.

Would you take the offer? Certainly not!!!

And yet that is exactly the opportunity that a stammerer over six years of age has to outgrow his trouble.

Dr. Leonard Keene Hirschberg, the medical writer, whose suggestions appear daily in a large list of newspapers, has this to say about the possibility of outgrowing stammering:

"Often when the attention of careless and reckless fatalistic relatives is attracted to a child's stammering, they labor under the mistaken illusion that the child 'will outgrow it.' A more harmful doctrine has never been perpetuated than the one contained in that stock phrase. As a matter of experience, speech troubles are not 'outgrown.' They become 'ingrown.' If not corrected at first they go from bad to worse. So firmly rooted and ingrained into the child's habits does stuttering become that with every hour's growth the chance for a cure becomes farther and farther removed."

This statement from Dr. Hirschberg is a straight-forward, practical and common-sense view of the subject.

The belief that the child will outgrow the malady often springs out of the tendency of the stammerer to be better and worse by turns, a condition which is fully described and explained in the chapter on the Intermittent Tendency. There is always present in any case of stammering the opportunity for a cessation of the trouble for a short period of time. The visible condition is changeable and it is this particular aspect of the disorder that renders it deceptive and dangerous, for many, who find themselves talking fairly well for a short period, believe that they are on the road to relief, whereas they are simply in a position where their trouble is about to return upon them in greater force than ever.

From the nature of the impediment--lack of co-ordination between the brain and the organs of speech--stammering cannot be outgrown --no more so than the desire to eat or to talk or to sleep.

Back of that statement, there is a very sound scientific reason that explains why stammering cannot be outgrown. Stammering is destructive. It tears down but cannot build up. Every time the stammerer attempts to speak and fails, the failure tears out a certain amount of his power-of-will. And since it is impossible for him to speak fluently except on rare occasions, this loss of will-power and confidence takes place every time he attempts to speak, so that with each successive failure, his power to speak correctly becomes steadily lessened. The case of a stammerer might be compared to a road in which a deep rut has been worn. Each time a wagon passes through this rut, it becomes deeper. The stammerer has no more chance of outgrowing his trouble than the road has of outgrowing the rut.

Dr. Alexander Melville Bell recognizes the absolute certainty of the progress of stammering and the impossibility of outgrowing the difficulty, when he states in his work, PRINCIPLES OF SPEECH (page 234):

"If the stammerer or stutterer were brought under treatment before the spasmodic habit became established, his cure would be much easier than after the malady has become rooted in his muscular and nervous system."

To the stammerer or stutterer or the parents of a stammering child, experience brings no truer lesson than this: Stammering cannot be outgrown; danger lurks behind delay.

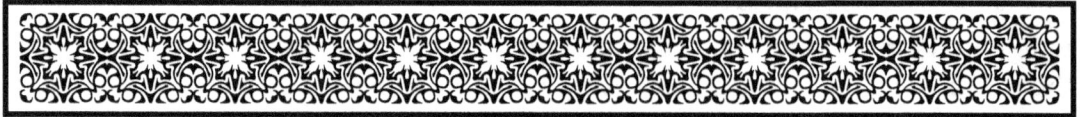

CHAPTER VII
THE EFFECT ON THE MIND

I t is hardly necessary to describe to the stammerer who has passed beyond the first stage of his trouble the effect of stammering on the mind. Most any sufferer in the second or third stages of the malady has experienced for very brief periods the sensation of thoughts slipping away from him and of pursuing or attempting to pursue those thoughts for some seconds without success, finally to find them returning like a flash.

The stammerer who recalls such an incident will remember the feelings of lassitude or momentary physical exhaustion, as well as the feeling of weakness which followed the lapse-of-thought. This mental flurry is but an indication of a mental condition known as Thought-Lapse, which may result from long-continued stammering, especially a case which has been allowed to progress into the Chronic or Advanced Stage.

A CASE OF APHASIA: One writer, in citing instances of thought- lapse, or aphasia, tells of the case of a man unable to recall the name of any object until it was repeated for him. A knife, for instance, placed on the table before him, brought no mental image of the word representing the object, yet if the word "knife" were spoken for him, he would immediately say, "Oh, yes, it is a knife."

A chapter could be filled with instances of this sort, but I shall not attempt to quote further any of the symptoms of aphasia in a stammerer, for in cases that become so far advanced, there is considerable question as to the possibility of bringing about a cure. I say this, notwithstanding the fact that my experience with students having this tendency has been very satisfactory indeed.

Cases of unreasoning despondency, which result in the stammerer's desire to take his own life, are so numerous as hardly to require comment. Very frequently you see in some of the large metropolitan papers an account of a suicide resulting from a nervous and mental condition brought on by stuttering and stammering. This condition seems to be very marked in the cases of stammerers between the ages of twelve and twenty, records showing that most of the suicides of stammerers are persons between those ages.

The intense mental strain, the extreme nervous condition, the continual worry and fear cannot fail, sooner or later, to have its effect upon the mind. This is clear to any stammerer, who is familiar with the mental condition brought about by the first few hours of one of his periods of recurrence. Another case where the mental strain is extremely great is that of the synonym stammerer --the mentally alert individual who, in order to prevent the outward appearance of stammering, is continually searching for synonyms or less difficult words to take the place of those which he cannot speak. This continual searching for synonyms results in a nervous tension that is sure to tell on the mental faculties sooner or later, and I have found, in examining many thousands of cases, that the synonym stammerer is usually in a more highly nervous state than any other type.

MENTAL STRAIN EVENTUALLY TELLS: The effect of stuttering or stammering on the sufferer's concentration is very marked. The sufferer notes an inability to concentrate his mind on any subject for any length of time, finds it impossible to pursue an education with any degree of success or to follow any business which requires close attention and careful work.

The power-of-will is also affected and the stammerer notes an inability to put through the things which he starts and which require the exercise of will power to bring to a successful conclusion.

A diagnosis of insanity is sometimes made in the case of a stammerer in the advanced stages of his malady, while in other instances the mental aberration takes the form of a hallucination of some sort, as in the case of the boy who was of the belief that he was continually being followed.

But regardless of what form is taken by the mental disorder resulting from stammering, such cases are almost invariably found to have long since passed into the incurable stage, although positive statements as to the individual's condition should not be made, as a rule, without a thorough diagnosis having first been made.

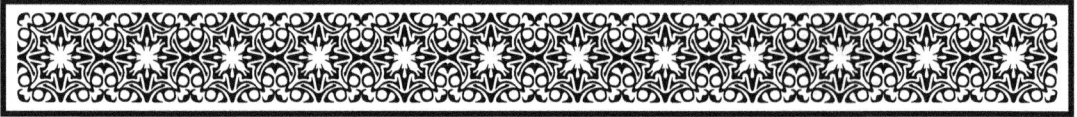

CHAPTER VIII
THE EFFECTS ON THE BODY

The effect of stammering or stuttering upon the physical structure is problematical. In some cases examined, a noticeable lack of vitality has been found, together with an almost total loss of active appetite, a marked inclination toward insomnia and a generally debilitated condition resulting from the nervous strain and continued fear brought on by the speech disorder.

In other cases, it has been found that the health was but little affected and that there was no marked departure from normal.

The physical condition of the stammerer is the result of many factors. If plenty of fresh air and exercise is supplied, and the mind is well-employed so that the worry over the trouble does not disturb the stammerer, then the chances for being in a normal physical condition are good.

On the other hand, the boy of studious disposition, who is somewhat of a bookworm, keeps close to the house and does not play with other children of his age, will probably find time for much introspection, and on this account, as well as on account of the lack of fresh air and exercise, will probably be in a physical condition that of itself demands careful attention.

It has been found in examinations of stammerers and stutterers, however, that they are usually of below normal chest expansion and that the health, while not particularly bad, is subject to a great improvement as a result of the proper treatment for stammering.

Charles Kingsley, the noted English divine and writer, and himself a stammerer many years ago, has the following to say regarding the effect of stammering on the body: "Continual depression of spirit wears out body as well as mind. The lungs never act rightly, never oxygenate the blood sufficiently. The vital energy continually directed to the organs of speech and there used up in the miserable spasm of mis-articulation cannot feed the rest of the body; and the man too often becomes thin, pale, flaccid, with contracted chest, loose ribs and bad digestion. I have seen a boy of twelve stunted, thin as a ghost and with every sign of approaching consumption. I have seen that boy a few months after being cured, upright, ruddy, stout, eating heartily and beginning to grow faster than he had ever grown in his life. I never knew a single case in which the health did not begin to improve then and there."

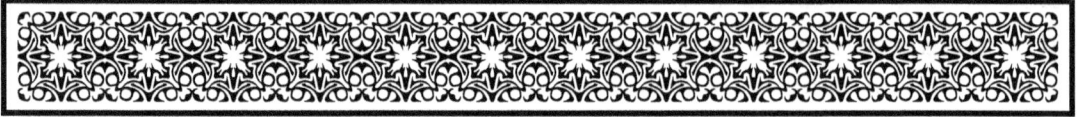

CHAPTER IX
DEFECTIVE SPEECH IN CHILDREN

(1) THE PRE-SPEAKING PERIOD

From the standpoint of speech development, the life of any person between the time of birth and the age of twenty-one years, may be divided into four periods as follows:

> From Birth to Age 2--PRE-SPEAKING PERIOD.
> Age 2 to Age 6--FORMATIVE-SETTING PERIOD
> Age 6 to Age 11--SPEECH-SETTING PERIOD
> Age 11 to Age 20--ADOLESCENT PERIOD

This chapter will deal only with the first period of the child's speech-development, beginning with birth and taking the child up to his second year. The speech disorders of the later periods will be taken up in the three following chapters.

THE PRE-SPEAKING PERIOD: This is the period between the time of birth and the age of 2, and takes the child up to the time of the first spoken word. This does not mean, of course, that no child speaks before the age of 2, for many children have made their first trials at speaking at as early an age as 15 months, and many begin to talk by the time they are a year and a half old. At the age of two, however, not only the precocious child but the child of slower-than-average development should be able to talk in at least brief, disjointed monosyllables.

Before taking up the possibility of a child exhibiting symptoms of defective speech with the first utterance, let us familiarize ourselves with the fundamentals underlying the production of the first spoken words.

The mother, who for months, perhaps, has been listening with eager interest and fond anticipation for her child's first word to be spoken, has little comprehension of the vast amount of education and training which the infant has absorbed in order to perfect this first small utterance. Months have been spent in listening to others, in taking in sounds and recalling them, in impressing them upon the memory by constant repetition, until finally after a year and a half, or more, perhaps, the circuit is completed and the first word is put down as history.

ASSOCIATION OF IDEAS: It must be remembered that perfect co- ordination of speech is the result of many mental images, not of one. In saying the word "salt," for instance, you have a graphic mental picture of what salt looks like; a second picture of what the word sounds like; a "motor-memory" picture of the successive muscle movements necessary to the formation of the word; another picture that recalls the taste of salt, and still another that recalls the movements of the hand necessary to write the word.

These pictures all hinging upon the word "salt" were gradually acquired from the time you began to observe. You tasted salt. You saw it at the same time you tasted it. There you see was an association of two ideas. Thereafter, when you saw salt, you not only recognized it by sight, but your brain recalled the taste of salt, without the necessity of your really tasting it. Or, on the other hand, if you had shut your eyes and someone had put salt on your tongue, the taste in that case would have recalled to your mind the graphic picture of the appearance of salt.

As you grew older and learned to speak, your vocal organs imitated the sound of the word "salt" as you heard it expressed by others and thus you learned to speak that word. At that stage, your brain was capable of calling up three mental pictures--an auditory picture, or a picture of the sound of the word; a graphic or visual picture, or a picture of the appearance of salt and a third, which we have called a motor-memory picture, which represents the muscular movements necessary to speak the word. A little later on, after you had gone to school and learned to write, you added to these pictures a fourth, the movements of the hand necessary to write the word "salt."

At the sight of the mother, a child may, for instance, be heard to say the word "Mom" while at the sight of the pet dog whose name is "Dot," be heard to say "Dot" in his childish way.

Here we have the first example in this child of the association of ideas. The child has heard, repeatedly, the word "Mama" used in conjunction with the appearance of the smiling face of his mother. Thus has the child acquired the habit of associating the word "Mama" with that face--and the sight of the countenance after a time recalls the sound of the associated word. Thus a visual image of the mother transmitted to the child through the medium of the eye, links up a train of thought that finally results in the child's attempt to say "Mama."

To take another example of the association of ideas or the co- ordination of mental images necessary to the production of speech, let us suppose, for instance, that the child has been in the habit of petting the dog and hearing him called by name "Dot" at the same time. Now, if the dog be placed out of the child's sight and yet in a position where the hand of the child can reach and pet him in a familiar way, this sense of touch, like the sense of sight, will set up a train of thought that results in the child making his childish attempt to speak the name of the dog "Dot."

In other words the excitation of any sensory organs sets up a series of sensory impulses which are transmitted along the sensory nerve fibres to the brain, where they are referred to the cerebellum or filing case, locating a set of associated impulses which travel outward from the motor area of the brain and result in the actions, or series of actions, which are necessary to produce a word.

It will make the action of the brain clearer if the reader will remember the sensory nerve fibres as those carrying messages only TO the brain, while the motor nerve fibres carry messages only FROM the brain.

To make still clearer this association of ideas so necessary to the production of speech, suppose this same child hears the word "Dot" spoken in his presence. He will, in all probability, begin to repeat the word, and to search diligently for his pet dog. Thus it will be seen that in this case the sound of the dog's name has stirred up a train of mental images, one of these being a visual image of the dog himself, causing the child to look about in search for him.

HOW WE LEARN TO TALK: We learn to talk, therefore, purely by observation and imitation. Observation is here used in a broad sense and means not only SEEING but SENSING, such as sensing by smelling, touching or tasting. The child imitates the sounds he hears and if these sounds emanate from those afflicted with defective utterance, then it follows that the initial utterance of the child will be likewise defective.

SOURCE OF THE FIRST WORD: The first spoken word of the child usually finds its source in some name or word repeatedly spoken in the child's presence. It is not usual that this first word is marked by a defective utterance and if such should be the case, then it is safe to say that this faulty utterance can be traced back to the imitation of some member of the family, or some child who has been permitted to talk to the child in his pre-speaking period. There is little to be gained by tracing the first word back, for no very profound conclusion can safely be registered with such a basis, for no matter what the word be and no matter whether it be correctly or imperfectly enunciated, it is the result of imitation.

There may be two exceptions to this, however, one being the case of a child with a physical defect in the organs of speech and the other that of a child who has inherited from the parents a predisposition to stammer or stutter. These exceptions, however, are so rare as to hardly require consideration. In the first (that of a physical defect) it is hardly probable that an organic defect would manifest itself in the form of stuttering or stammering, but rather in some other form of defective utterance. In the case of the inherited predisposition to stutter or stammer, there is always the question which has contributed more largely to the defective utterance--the inherited predisposition or the association with others who speak in a faulty manner.

ADVICE TO PARENTS: It is very essential that from the very beginning of the period of the recording of suggestion, the child is shown the correct and customary utterance with the best method of its accomplishment. The child should not be subjected to constant repetitions of phonetic defects, imperfect utterance or speech disorders of any sort. The child who hears none but perfect speech is not liable to speak imperfectly, or at least not so liable as the child who hears wrong methods of talking in use at all times, for this last cannot escape the effects of his environment.

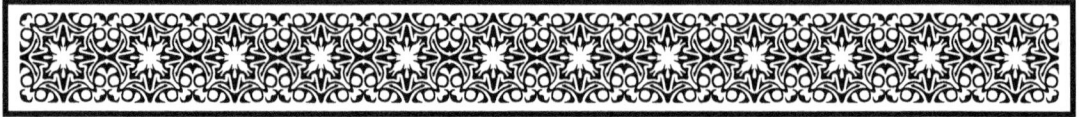

CHAPTER X
DEFECTIVE SPEECH IN CHILDHEN

(2) THE FORMATIVE PERIOD

The period in a child's speech development dating from the second year and up to the sixth, is called the Formative Period, for the reason that this is the time when the child is busy learning new words, acquiring new habits of speech, co-ordinating and learning properly to associate the flood of ideas which overwhelm the child-mind in this period.

The child-vocabulary at this time is but an echo of the vocabulary of the home. The words that have been used most frequently there are most strongly impressed upon the child-mind. The names he has heard, the objects he has seen, the applications of speech-ideas-- these alone are now in his mind. This condition is inevitable since the child must learn to speak by imitation--and, since he has had no source of word--pictures other than the home, he must have acquired facility in the use of only those words he has had an opportunity to hear.

Former President Wilson, whose faultless diction, remarkable fluency of expression and discriminating choice of words, made him a master speaker and writer, attributed his facility to the training he received in the home of his father, a minister, where the children were constantly encouraged in the use of correct English and in the broadening and enrichment of their store of words.

From the form of simple child-speech, made up often of monosyllables or of a few brief and easy sentences, the child must now evolve a more complicated form of thought-expression, with the use of connectives, descriptions and a finer gradation of color than heretofore.

This process may be materially aided by the parent by the repetition of the child's own utterances, proving to the child that these are correct, that he is being understood and giving him confidence to venture further out in his attempts at speech amplification. This encouragement of the child-mind in its attempts to speak is so important that it is worth while to give some simple examples of what is meant, in order that the point may be clearly understood. Let us take, first, the example of a mother who, from some cause, allows herself to be of a nervous and irritable disposition. The small child may say, "Mam--ma, I want a tooky." The mo-ther, either through indifference or through habit, says, "You want WHAT?" This, first of all, is like a dash of cold water to the child in his uncertain state of mind as to the correctness of his utterance. The child repeats, "I want a tooky," and in all probability gets the further inquiry, "You want a TOOKY--what's that?" which undermines the child's confidence in himself and in his ability to talk.

On the other hand, the mother who understands the needs of the child from a speech-forming standpoint will not insist on the child repeating the word time after time as if it was not understood. She will strive hard to understand the first time, even though the expression is imperfect and difficult of interpretation, and her nimble mind having figured out what it is that the child desires, will say, "Baby wants a cooky?" Here the child, in his comparatively new occupation of talking, finds a deal of delight in knowing that his words have been properly comprehended and feels a new confidence in his ability to express thoughts--which confidence, by the way, is essential to normal speech development in the child. It has the further effect of correcting the tendency of faulty utterance, and in time will result in the complete eradication of the natural tendency to "baby-talk" which is too often encouraged and aided by the habit of parents in REPEATING THE BABY-TALK. In no case, should defective utterances be repeated, no matter how "cute" the utterance may seem at the time. Many speak indistinctly throughout their entire life simply because of the habit of their parents in repeating baby-talk, thus confirming incorrect images of numerous words.

SPEECH DISORDERS IN THE FORMATIVE PERIOD: The Formative Period may mark the beginning of a speech disorder and in many instances chronic cases of stuttering and stammering may be traced to a simple disorder which first manifested itself in the ages between 2 and 6.

Speech disorders arising in this period may be traced to any one of a number of causes. In a child of five, for instance, the diagnostician would look for evidences of an inherited tendency to stammer or stutter; he would look also for circumstances which would show that the child had acquired defective utterance through mimicry of others similarly afflicted or through the unconscious imitation of the defective speech of those immediately about him.

Failing to find any hereditary tendency to a speech defect or any evidence that the disorder had been acquired by imitation or mimicry, the next step would be to determine whether or not the trouble had been caused by disease or injury.

As explained in Chapter III, the diseases of childhood, such as Whooping Cough, Scarlet Fever, Diphtheria, Acute Chorea, Infantile Cerebral Palsy and Infantile Paralysis are frequently the cause of stuttering or stammering, and a history showing a record of these diseases would result in a very careful examination for the purpose of determining if they had resulted in a form of defective utterance.

ADVICE TO PARENTS: But whatever the cause of the trouble, care should be taken to see that it grows no worse and every attempt should be made to eradicate it at this early stage. Like a fire, speech disorders in their early stages are insignificant compared to their future progress and can be much more readily eradicated then than later. Inasmuch as a child of less than eight years is hardly old enough to undertake institutional treatment successfully, it behooves the parent of the stammering or stuttering child to render what home assistance is possible, during this period. The old adage, tried and true, that "An ounce of prevention is worth a pound of cure" is never more correctly applied than here. A few simple suggestions may aid in preventing the trouble from progressing rapidly to a serious stage, even though these suggestions do not eradicate the disorder altogether.

First of all, the child should be kept in the very best possible physical condition. This means, too, plenty of fresh air and sunshine, without which any child is less than physically fit.

It is important that the child be not allowed to associate with others who stammer or stutter, or who have any form of speech disorder. Imitation or mimicry, as heretofore stated, is the most prolific cause of speech trouble and to place a child who stammers or stutters in the company of an older person similarly afflicted, is to invite a serious form of the disorder.

Nervousness, while not the cause of speech disorder, is an aggravant of the trouble and should be avoided. The child should not be allowed to engage in anything which has a tendency to make him nervous or highly excited. Such a condition will aggravate the speech trouble, make it worse and tend to fix it more firmly in the child.

Furthermore, parents should not scold or berate the child because he stammers or stutters. No child stammers or stutters because he wants to, but because he has not the power to control his speech organs. In other words, the child cannot help himself--and scolding and harsh words simply cause confusion and dejection which in turn react to make a more serious condition.

THE CHANCES FOR OUTGROWING: The author's examination and diagnosis of more than 20,000 cases of speech disorders has revealed the fact that at this period in the life of the child afflicted with stammering or stuttering, slightly less than 1 percent. outgrow the difficulty. With proper parental care it might be possible to increase this percentage, perhaps double it, but this should hardly be called "outgrowing." In the mind of the average person, the expression "outgrowing his stammering" means that the stammerer has been able to go ahead without giving the slightest heed to his trouble and that it has, by some magical process, ceased to exist. This is a fallacy. Stammering and stuttering are both destructive and progressive and no amount of indifference will result in relief--but on the other hand, will terminate in a more malignant type of the disorder. It IS true, however, that more care on the part of the parent in looking after the formation of speech habits in the Pre-Speaking and Formative Periods of the child's speech development, would result in fewer cases of chronic stammering and stuttering in later life.

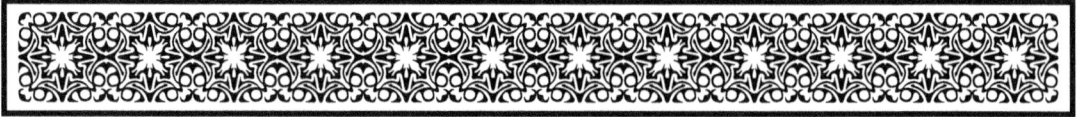

CHAPTER XI
DEFECTIVE SPEECH IN CHILDREN

(3) THE SPEECH-SETTING PERIOD

The period from the age of 6 to the age of 11 (inclusive) is in truth the Speech-Setting Period, for it is at this time that the child's speech habits become more or less fixed, and his vocabulary, while constantly developing, manifests tendencies which may be traced through into the later life of the adult.

This Speech-Setting Period marks two very important events in the speech development of the child. First, it marks the period of second dentition or the time when the milk-teeth are "shed" and the new and permanent teeth take their place. This is a critical period and statistics show that there is a marked increase in speech disorders at this time. The second event of importance, both to child and to parents, is the beginning of the work in school. It must be remembered that heretofore the child has been under the watchful care of the parents during most of his hours, while now, with the beginning of his work in school, he is having his first small taste of facing the world alone--even if only for a little while each day.

Regardless of the attitude which the child takes toward his work in school, this work presents new problems and new possibilities of danger from a standpoint of speech development. A slight defect in utterance which at home is passed over from long familiarity, is the subject of ridicule and laughter at school. For the first time in the child-life, the stammering or stuttering youngster may experience the awful feeling of being laughed at and made fun of, without exactly knowing why. He will have to face the questions of his thoughtless companions who will attempt to make him talk merely for the sake of entertaining themselves. To the child who stutters or stammers, this is torture in its worst form. The humiliation and disgrace which the stammering child must undergo on the way to school, in the school-yard and on the way home again, is a tremendous force in the life of the youngster--a force which may seriously impede his mental development, his physical welfare and his progress in school. He finds himself unlike others, deficient in some respect and yet not realizing the exact nature of his deficiency or understanding why it should be a deficiency. He stands up to recite with a constantly increasing fear of failure in his heart and unless he is fortunate enough to have a teacher who understands, is apt to fare poorly at her hands, also. Even in the case of the teacher who does understand the child's difficulty and consequently permits written instead of oral recitations, there is a constant feeling of inability on the part of the child, a knowledge of being less-whole than those about him, which saps the self-confidence so necessary to proper mental development and normal progress. He furthermore misses much of the value of the studies that he pursues, for, as a noted educator has said, "In order for a child to remember and fix clearly in his own mind the things he studies, those things must be repeated in oral recitation." And this the stammering or stuttering child cannot do.

SENDING STAMMERING CHILDREN TO SCHOOL: With these facts in mind, the question arises as to whether it is ever policy to send a stammering or stuttering child to school, knowing that he is afflicted with a speech-disorder. In the first place the parents who send a stammering child to school exhibit a careless disregard for the rights of others and a further disregard for the many children who must, of a necessity, associate with this stammering child, with all the consequent dangers of infection by imitation or mimicry. Speech defects of a remediable nature among school children could be materially reduced by refusing to allow children so afflicted to play or in any way associate with the others who talk normally.

Aside, however, from the question of the parents' obligation to society and to the children of others (which should be, in the end, a means of protection for their own children, as well) there is the bigger and more selfish aspect of the question, viz.: the effect on the child himself.

No better suggestion can be given than that contained in "The Habit of Success" by Luther H. Gulick, who says: "If you take a child that is really mentally subnormal and put him in school with normal children, he cannot do well no matter how hard he tries. He tries again and again and fails. Then he is scolded and punished, kept after school and held up to the ridicule of the teacher and other students. When he goes out on the playground, he cannot play with the vigor and skill and force of other children. In the plays, he is not wanted on either side; he is always 'it' in tag. So he soon acquires the presentment that he is going to fail no matter what he does, that he cannot do as the others do and that there is no use in trying. So he gives up trying. He quits.

"That is the largest element in the lives of the feeble-minded-- that conviction that they cannot do like others, and is the first thing they must overcome if they are to be helped. There is no hope whatever of growth, as long as they foresee they are going to fail."

The futility of trying to "cram" an education into a subnormal child has never been better expressed than in the statement quoted above. There is nothing to be gained by insisting that a child who is ill, attend school--and it should be remembered that so far as school is concerned, the child who stutters or stammers is just as ill as the one with the measles, save that the illness of the stammering or stuttering child is chronic and persistent, while that of the other is temporary.

CHANCES FOR OUTGROWING AT THIS AGE: The opportunities for the stammering or stuttering child to outgrow his trouble are about five times as great in the Formative Period, between the ages of 2 and 6, as they are in the Speech-Setting Period, from 6 to 11. In the former, as previously explained, statistics show that about 1 per cent.--or one in a hundred--outgrow their trouble before the age of 6, while after this age the percentage drops to one-fifth of one per cent, or about one person in every five hundred, which is a very small chance indeed.

In speaking of the tendency of parents to wait in the hope that speech disorders will be outgrown, Walter B. Swift, A.B., S.B., M.D., has this to say:

"This suggestion may frequently be offered, even by the physician. Many people say, 'Let the case alone and it will outgrow its defect.' No treatment could be more foolish than this. No advice could be more ill-advised; no suggestion could show more ignorance of the problems of speech. Such advisers are ignorant of the harm they are doing and the amount of mental drill of which they are depriving the pupil. Nor do they know at all whether or not the case will ever 'outgrow' its defect. In brief, this advice is without foundation, without scientific backing, and should never be followed."

ADVICE TO PARENTS: Parents of children between the ages of 6 and 11 who stammer or stutter, should follow out the suggestions given in the previous chapter, with the idea of removing the difficulty in its incipiency if possible, or at least of preventing its progress. If by the time the child is eight years of age, the defective utterance remains, this fact is proof that the speech disorder is of a form that will not yield to the simple methods possible under parental treatment at home and the child should be immediately placed under the care of an expert whose previous knowledge and experience insures his ability to correct the defective utterance quickly and permanently.

In all cases after the age of 8, the matter should be taken firmly in hand. There should be no dilly-dallying, no foolish belief in the possibility of outgrowing the trouble, for whatever chances once existed are now past. First of all, the child's case should be diagnosed by an expert with the idea of ascertaining the exact nature of the speech disorder, the probable progress of the trouble, the present condition, the curability of the case and the possibilities for early relief. A personal diagnosis should be secured where possible, but when this cannot be brought about, a written description and history of the case should enable the capable diagnostician of speech defects to diagnose the case in a very thorough manner. The result of this diagnosis should be set down in the form of a report in order that the parent may have a permanent record of the child's condition and may be able to take the proper steps for the eradication of the speech disorder. With this information as to the child's case in hand, parents should be guided by the advice of Alexander Melville Bell, one of the greatest speech specialists of his age, who said:

"Stuttering and Hesitation are stages through which the stammerer generally passes before he reaches the climax of his difficulty, and if he were brought under treatment before the spasmodic habit became established, his cure would be much more easy than after the malady has become rooted in his muscular and nervous system."

Truly may it be said of the stammering child at this period, that "There is a tide in the affairs of men, which taken at the flood, leads on to fortune; omitted, all the voyage of their life is bound in shallows and in miseries."

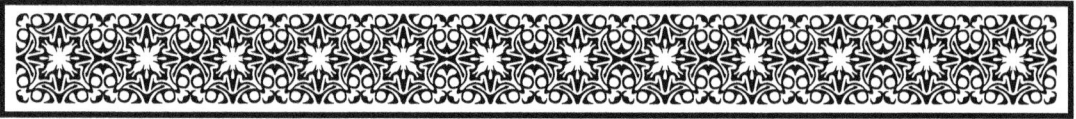

CHAPTER XII
THE SPEECH DISORDERS OF YOUTH

Youth, as we shall define it from the standpoint of the development of speech disorders, is the period from the age of 12 to the age of 20. From the twelfth to the twentieth year is a very critical period in the life of both the boy and the girl who stammers--a period which should have the watchfulness and care of the parent at every step. This is known as the period of adolescence and may be said to mark the time of a new birth, when both mind and body undergo vital changes. New sensations, many of them intense, arise, and new associations in the sense sphere are formed.

To the boy or girl passing through this stage of life, it is a period of new and unknown forces, emotions and feelings. It is a time of uncertainty. The sure-footed confidence of childhood gives way to the unsure, hesitating, questioning attitude of a mind filled with new and strange thoughts and a body animated by new and strange sensations.

These are the symptoms of a fundamental change, the outward manifestations of the passing from childhood to manhood or womanhood. This is childhood's equinoctial storm, marking the beginning of the second season of life's year. In this storm, it is the paramount duty of the parent to be a safe and ever-present pilot through the sea that to the captain of this craft is as uncharted as the route to the Indies in Columbus' day.

The revolution now taking place in both the mental and bodily processes results hi a lack of stability--an "unsettledness" that manifests itself in restlessness, nervousness, self-consciousness or morbidness, taking perhaps the form of a persistent melancholia or desire to be alone.

At this time in the life of the boy or girl, the possibilities for stuttering or stammering to secure a firm hold on their muscular and nervous system are very great. Next to the age of second dentition, children at the age of puberty are most susceptible to stammering or stuttering.

During adolescence, the annual rate of growth in height, weight and strength is increased and often doubled or more. The power of the diseases peculiar to childhood abates and the liability to the far more numerous diseases of maturity begins, so that with the liability to both it is not strange that this period is marked at the same time by increased morbidity.

The significant fact about stuttering in children as far as it relates to the period of adolescence, is that this stage marks the most pronounced susceptibility to the malady as well as the time during which it may most quickly pass into the chronic stage. Examinations show that the largest percentage of stutterers among boys was at the ages of eight, thirteen and sixteen, while the largest percentage among girls was at the ages of seven, twelve and sixteen--the earlier age of severity in girls being explained by the fact that the girl reaches a given state of maturity more quickly than a boy.

Parents of stammering or stuttering children between the ages of twelve and twenty, may well note with alarm the increasing nervousness, the hyper-sensitive feelings, the overpowering self- consciousness and the morbid tendencies which mark a state of mental depression, brooding and worry over troubles both real and fancied.

PERIOD OF MOST FREQUENT SUICIDE: Statistics gathered over a period of years indicate that the cases of suicide of stammering children occur at this time with greater frequency than at any other. Rarely has a case been found where a child has attempted to take his life before the age of 12 and seldom after the age of 20.

At frequent intervals there can be found in any of the large papers, a very brief note of the suicide of a child who had found life too much of a burden for him to bear and who, as a consequence, fell to brooding over his troubles and as the easiest way out of them, took his own life. A Chicago boy attempted suicide by inhaling gas, although he was discovered before it was too late. Another took his own life by shooting himself with a revolver given him some years ago as a birthday present; still another took poison as the easiest way out of his humiliation, embarrassment and despair.

The average age of these boys was about 16 1/2 years, which marks a period of intense self-consciousness and extreme sensitiveness of the youth to ridicule and disgrace.

TENDENCY TO RAPID PROGRESS: The condition of the young person between the ages of 12 and 20 can hardly be considered to be normal in any way. The physical processes are un-normal and are undergoing a change, and the mental faculties, too, are un- normal, overwhelmed as they are with new emotions and sensations. The nervous condition is marked by a much higher nervous irritability, which contributes to a condition most favorable for the rapid progress of the speech disorder, always easily aggravated by a subnormal physical, mental or nervous condition. Cases where the Intermittent Tendency is a pronounced characteristic are liable at this period to find the alternate periods of relief and recurrence to be more frequent than ever before and to note a marked tendency of their trouble to recur with constantly increasing malignancy. Cases that at the age of 11 or 12, for instance, might have been said to have been in an incipient state, have commonly been known at this age to pass through the successive intermediate stages of the trouble and become of a deep-seated and chronic nature in a surprisingly short period of time.

In some cases where the transition from a simple to the complex form of the difficulty takes place at this age, it is found that the disorder has passed beyond the curable stage, in which case, of course, nothing is left to the unfortunate stammerer but the prospects of a life of untold misery and torture, deprived of companionship, ostracized from society and debarred from participation in either business or the professions.

CHANCES OF OUTGROWING: The chances for outgrowing a speech disorder at this age are considerably less than at any other time in the previous life of the individual. The unbalanced general condition tends to make the stammerer more susceptible instead of less so. As previously explained, this period marks the time when speech disorders progress rapidly from bad to worse and, as a consequence, the chances for outgrowing diminished from 1 per cent, before the age of 6 to practically zero after the age of 12. SUGGESTIONS: There is little that can be said for the good of the young person at these ages. The time for home treatment is past. The simple suggestions offered for the assistance of those in the Formative or Speech-Setting Periods would be of little value here because the growth of the individual has made the eradication of the trouble quite improbable without a complete re-education along correct speech lines--best obtained from an institution devoting its efforts to that work. Whatever steps are taken, however, should be taken before the disorder has become rooted in the muscular and nervous system and before it has passed into the Chronic Stage.

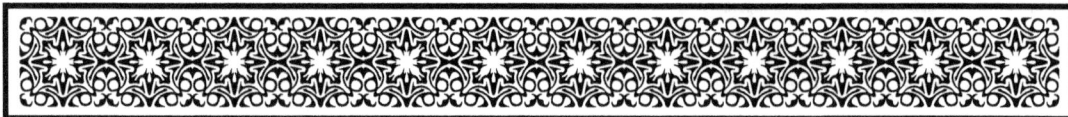

CHAPTER XIII
WHERE DOES STAMMERING LEAD?

In answering the question: "Where Does Stammering Lead?" nothing truer can be found than the words of a man who has stammered himself:

"What pen can depict the woefulness, the intensified suffering of the inveterate stammerer, confirmed, stereotyped in a malady seemingly worse than death? Are the afflictions, mental and physical, of the pelted, brow-beaten, downtrodden stutterer imaginary? Nonsense! There is not a word of truth in the idea. His sufferings all the time, day in and day out, at home and abroad, are real--intense--purgatorial. And none but those who have drunk the bitter cup to its dregs feel and know its death, death, double death! These afflicted ones die daily and the graves to them seem pleasant and delightful. The sufferings of the deaf and dumb are myths--but a drop in the ocean compared to what I endured! And who cared for me? Who? I wag the laughing stock, a subject of scoffing and ridicule, often. I could fill an octavo with the miseries I endured from early childhood till the elapsement of forty summers."

Thus does the Rev. David F. Newton, himself a stammerer for forty years, speak of stammering and stuttering and its effects. And Charles Kingsley, a noted English divine and author who stammered, paints the stammerer's future in words of experience that no stammerer should ever forget:

"The stammerer's life is a life of misery, growing with his growth and deepening as his knowledge of life and his aspirations deepen. One comfort he has, truly, that his life will not be a long one. Some may smile at this assertion; let them think for themselves. How many old people have they ever heard stammer! I have known but two. One is a very slight ease, the other a very severe one. He, a man of fortune, dragged on a very painful and pitiful existence-- nervous, decrepit, asthmatic--kept alive by continual nursing. Had he been a laboring man, he would have died thirty years sooner than he did."

To the man who has never been through the suffering that results from stammering or who has never been privileged to watch the careers of stammerers and stutterers over a period of years, these final results of stammering seem impossible. The inexperienced observer can only ask in wonder: "How can stammering or stuttering bring a man or woman to these depths of despair?"

To the stammerer who has but begun to taste the sorrows of a stammerer's life these effects of stammering appear to be the ultimate result of an UNUSUAL case-- never the inevitable result of his own trouble.

Doubtless if Charles Kingsley were with us today, he could look back and tell us of the day when he, too, was sure that stammering was but a trifle. He, too, could point out the tune when he felt that sometime, somehow, his stammering would magically depart and leave him free to talk as others talked. And yet, having gone down the road through a long lif e of usefulness, Kingsley's is the voice of a mature experience which says to every stammerer: "Beware--there are pitfalls ahead!" And this man is right.

RESULTS OF STAMMERING: Experience proves that the results of continued stammering or stuttering are definite and positive, and that they are inevitable. Stammering is known to be at the root of many troubles. It causes nervousness, self-consciousness and sometimes brings about a mental condition bordering on complete mental breakdown. It causes mental sluggishness, dissipates the power-of-concentration, weakens the power of will, destroys ambition and stands between the sufferer and an education.

There is no affliction more annoying or embarrassing to its victim than stammering. No matter how bright the intellect may be, if the tongue is unable easily and quickly to formulate the words expressing thought, the individual is held back in business and is debarred from the pleasures of social and home life.

Stammering is a drawback to children in school. To be unable to recite means failure. It means humiliation. It means disgrace in the eyes of the other pupils. And finally, it means valuable time wasted--not in getting an education--but in suffering untold misery in TRYING to get one--and failing.

A boy fourteen years of age, who has failed to advance in school, and who finds stammering a handicap of serious proportions, tells me:

"I am fourteen years old and only in the fifth grade. I am afraid to recite because of my stuttering, and because of my not reciting when my teachers call on me, I am getting low marks in school and do not know if I will ever get through."

One mother writes:

"My little girl will not go to Sunday School because she does not like the other children to look at her so straight when she stammers."

A boy says:

"I am thirteen years old and in school. I am afraid to recite because of my stuttering; and because of my not reciting I get low average in studies."

Another boy told me:

"I am now in the third year of my high school course. On the first day of the term I went to school, I made sueh a miserable thing of myself that I quit. The school superintendent and principal saw me when I came back the second day as I was carrying my books out. Of course they stopped me and I made an explanation. I couldn't tell any of the new teachers my name. It was impossible to make any kind of a recitation. I was introduced to all of my teachers and have been STUMBLING ALONG ever since with grades anywhere from 0 to 60."

A SOCIAL DRAWBACK: No stammerer but knows that his malady marks him for the half-suppressed smiles of thoughtless people and the unkind remarks of those who really know nothing of the suffering which these unkind remarks occasion. It is true, but unfortunate, that the stammerer is not wanted in any social gathering, he can provide no entertainment, save at his own expense, and of all people he is most ill at ease when out among others.

A young lady writes:

"Mr. Bogue, I would give one of my eyes to get rid of stammering. That is all I am after. Please excuse this awful writing. I AM SO NERVOUS I CAN HARDLY GET THE PEN INTO THE INK BOTTLE."

Here is a letter from one man:

"I am 36 years old, and have stammered for 28 years. I don't stammer so bad, but just bad enough to spoil my life. I always have to take a back seat in company. I belong to three lodges, but I do not take part in any of them because I am afraid they will ask me to take part in the order. It would make me feel cheap. I have often felt like committing suicide, but I would pull my nerves together and make the best of it again. I am now a janitor at a school."

HOPELESS IN BUSINESS: There is not a young man stammerer in this whole country who would not work night and day to be cured of stammering if he realized the hopelessness of trying to be a success in a business way, handicapped by stammering, unable to talk fluently, clearly and intelligently.

A man says:

"I am 33 years old and single. I have stammered ever since I was a child. It has made me nervous. At my age it is very embarrassing to me to stutter. I kept getting more nervous from year to year, and finally I have had to give up my position. I was a long-hand biller for ten years, but I am now troubled with writer's cramp and unable to do much. I can't get a clerk's job because of my stuttering."

And here is another--a man grown, who too late realized the futility of trying to get an education while yet handicapped by stammering. He said, a while back:

"I must say my stammering has spoiled my life and robbed me of a successful career. I would give much if my parents had sent me to be cured of stammering when a boy, instead of trying as they did to educate me."

STAMMERER APPEARS ILLITERATE: No matter how great the stammerer's knowledge may be, he often appears to be illiterate simply because he is unable to express himself in words. His knowledge is locked up by his infirmity, the same as though he had a steel band drawn over his mouth and fastened with a padlock which he is unable to unlock for want of a proper key. The man with the locked-up knowledge is under as great a handicap as the man without knowledge.

A man who had a chance to be a big success in business, had he not stammered, says:

"Stammering is the cause of all my trouble. My earlier associates have shunned me for several years, and I have sought the worst class of dives and the lowest kind of companions, where I was reasonably certain that I would not come in contact with those with whom I had associated in earlier years. My eyes are wet with tears--tears of remorse and regret--because I see no chance in life for me now."

The stammerer who thinks that success comes to the man who stammers--who believes that the business world is willing to put up with anything less than fluent speech, should read this heart- broken letter from a young man:

"I am a bookkeeper, and dearly love my work, but am afraid that I am going to have to give it up because my speech is getting worse, and I have noticed that the boss has mentioned it to me a couple of times now, and it almost breaks my heart to know that my position is going to get away from me. No one realizes how much one suffers, and I'm afraid I'm going to break down with nervous prostration soon. When one day is over with me, I wonder how I am going to get through with the next one."

What are the results of stammering? Should anyone ask that question, I could point to instances in my own experience that would prove that almost every undesirable condition of human existence may be the result of stammering. I have seen young men who are business failures, dejected, hopeless, drifting along, men who in early years were intellectual giants, and who before their death were mere children in mental power, because they allowed stammering to destroy every valuable faculty they possessed.

I could point to children whom stammering had held back almost from the time they began to talk--give cases of young men depressed, embarrassed, unsuccessful, because they stammer--cite instances of all the worth-while things in life turned from the path of a young woman because she stammered.

Yet in the past, not one of these knew what was coming. Not one realized where the trail was leading. No stammerer can of himself see into the future. But he can, at least, look into the future of others, who, like himself, are stammerers, and avoid the pitfalls into which they have fallen and save himself the mistakes they have made.

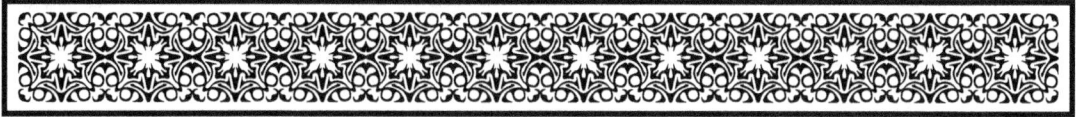

PART III
THE CURE OF STAMMERING AND STUTTERING

CHAPTER I
CAN STAMMERING BEALLY BE CURED?

It has only been a few years since the impression was abroad that stammering was incurable. Not a particle of hope was held out to the afflicted individual that any semblance of a cure was possible by any method. This erroneous idea that stammering could not be cured grew up in the mind of the average person as a result of one or all of the f ollowing conditions:

1st--The inability of the stammerer to cure himself and his further inability to outgrow the trouble, (although he was repeatedly told that he would outgrow it) was the first reason that led to the foolish and totally unfounded belief that stammering could not be cured.

2nd--The principles of speech and the un-normal condition known as stammering have been surrounded with a great deal of mystery in the years gone by. The idea has been widely prevalent that the affliction was one sent by Providence as a punishment for some act committed by the sufferer or his forbears. This and many other ideas bordering upon superstition, are responsible, too, to a great degree for the belief that stammering is incurable.

3rd--Even if an attempt to cure stammering was made, this attempt was based upon the "supposition" that stammering was a physical trouble, due to some defect in the organs of speech. It followed that since no one was ever able to discover any physical defect, no one knew the true cause of the disorder, nor how to treat it successfully.

4th--Unfortunately there have been in the field a number of irresponsible charlatans, preying upon the stammerer with claims to cure, while in fact they knew little or nothing of the disorder, had never stammered themselves, nor had the slightest knowledge of the correct methods of procedure in the core of stammering. The failure of such as these to do any good led to a widespread belief that there was no successful method for the eradication of speech disorders.

From an experience covering more than twenty-eight years, during which time the author has corresponded with 210,000 persons who stammer and has personally met and diagnosed about 22,000 cases, it has been proved that all of these beliefs are fallacies of the worst character. Given any person who stutters or stammers and who has no organic defect and is as intelligent as the average child of eight years, it has been found that the Unit Method of Restoring Speech will eradicate the trouble at its source and by removing the cause, entirely remove the defective utterance.

THE STAMMERER'S CASE NOT HOPELESS: Stammerers should fix this fact firmly in mind: Stammering can be cured! There is hope, positive, definite hope for every case--this fact is based on every imaginable form of stuttering or stammering. It is not, in other words, a mere idle statement based on theory or guess-work, but a mathematical truth, taken from experience.

I recall very well the case of a man of 32 who came to me for help after five of the so-called schools for stammerers had failed to afford him any relief. Quite naturally this man was a confirmed skeptic. He did not believe that there was any cure for him. Anyone who had been through the trials that he had experienced would have felt the same way. But he placed himself under treatment, nevertheless, and in a few weeks' time, the Unit Method had restored him to perfect speech. He left entirely convinced that stammering could be cured, because it had been done in his own case which had so long seemed beyond all hope.

Many years afterward, he wrote a letter which I take the liberty of reproducing here for the encouragement and inspiration of everyone who is similarly afflicted and who feels as this man felt--that he is incurable:

"I tried to be cured of stammering at five different times by five different men at a total cost of more than one thousand dollars. None of them cnred me. Then I decided to try the Unit Method. Nine years ago I did so--a decision that I have never regretted. It waa evident that this method was based on a comprehensive knowledge of the art of speech. I am now a piano salesman and talk by the hour all day long; talk over the telephone perfectly; and many tell me that I speak more distinctly than the majority of people who have never stammered. I believe this is because I was taught through the Unit Method the very fundamentals of speech."

This man's case is typical of the hundreds of failures-to-cure which are responsible for the belief that stammering cannot be cured. The fact that he had made five separate attempts to be cured would, in the mind of the average man, establish the fact that stammering cannot be cured and yet it is seen that even in this extreme case, under the application of the proper scientific methods, the stammerer found freedom of speech without unusual difficulty and in a comparatively short time.

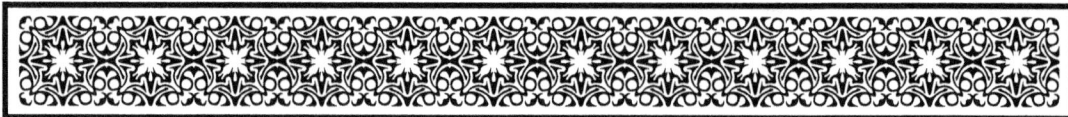

CHAPTER II
CASES THAT "CURE THEMSELVES"

Not infrequently from some source will be heard a story, many times retold, to the effect that "So-and-so" who stammered for many years has been cured--that the trouble has magically disappeared and that he stammers no longer.

What is the cause of this? What brings about such a miraculous cure?

The answer depends upon the case. Usually, the story is much more a story than a fact. Few indeed have been the stammerers who have ever actually heard the man stammer before "his trouble cured itself" and then heard him talk perfectly afterwards. Like the stories of haunted houses, there is nothing to substantiate the truth of the statement, there is no evidence by which the story may be checked up.

In the rare cases where the facts would seem to indicate the truth of the statement, it will be found that the person in question never really stammered--that his trouble was something else-- lalling, lisping, or some defect of speech that was mistaken for stammering or stuttering.

Another case of apparent miraculous cure is the case of the stammerer who, finding himself unable to say words beginning with certain letters, begins the practice of substituting easy sounds for those that are difficult and thus, provided he has only a slight case, leads many to believe that he talks almost perfectly. This fellow is known as the "Synonym Stammerer" and is usually a quick thinker and a ready "substituter-of-words." If he has stammered noticeably for some time until those in his vicinity have become acquainted with his affliction, and then discovers the plan of substituting easy sounds for hard ones, he may for a time conceal his impediment and lead certain of his friends to believe that he no longer stammers.

This "Synonym Stammerer" is storing up endless trouble for himself, however, for the mental strain of trying to remember and speak synonyms of hard words entails such a great drain upon his mind as to make it almost impossible to maintain the practice for any great length of tune. In this connection, let every stammerer be warned to avoid this practice of substitution of words. It is a seeming way out of difficulty sometimes, but you will find that you are only making your malady worse and laying up difficulties for yourself in the future.

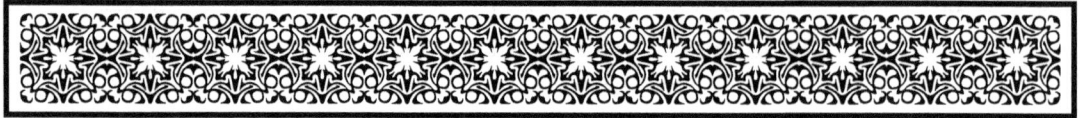

CHAPTER III
CASES THAT CANNOT BE CURED

In an experience in meeting stammerers and in curing stammering it is only natural to assume that I have come across certain cases which could not be cured. It is only natural, too, to expect that in such a wide experience it would be possible to determine what cases are incurable and why.

Cases of incurable speech impediments may be divided into seven classes:

    (1)--Those with organic defects;
    (2)--Those with diseased condition of the brain;
    (3)--Those who have postponed treatment until their malady
        has progressed so far into the chronic stage as to make
        treatment valueless;
    (4)--Those who refuse to obey instructions;
    (5)--Those who persist in dissipation, regardless of effects;
    (6)--Those of below normal intelligence;
    (7)--Those who will not make the effort to be cured.

Stutterers and stammerers whose trouble arises from an organic defect are so few as to be almost an exception, but where those cases exist, they must be regarded as incurable. The re- educational process used in the successful method of curing stuttering and stammering will not replace a defective organ of the body with a new one. It will not cure harelip or cleft palate, nor will it loosen the tongue of the child who has been hopelessly tongue-tied from birth.

A boy was brought to me some years ago by his parents in the hope that his speech trouble might be eradicated, but it was found upon examination that he had always been tongue-tied and that the deformity would not permit of the normal, natural movements of the tongue necessary to proper speaking. I immediately told the parents the unfortunate condition of their son and frankly stated that in his condition there was no possibility of my being able to help him.

DISEASED BRAIN: Taking up the second class--those who have a diseased condition of the brain--these cases, too, are very rare. I have met but a comparatively few. Where a lesion of the brain has occurred, and a distinct change has thus been brought about in the physical structure of that organ, an attempt to bring about a cure would be a waste of time--hopeless from the start.

THE PROCRASTINATORS: The third type of incurable cases is that of the stammerer or stutterer who, against all advice and experience, has persisted in the belief that his trouble would be outgrown and who has by this means allowed the disorder to progress so far into the chronic stage as to make treatment entirely without effect.

This type of incurable is very numerous. They usually start in childhood with a case of simple stuttering which, if treated then, could be eradicated quickly and easily. From this stage they usually pass into the trouble of a compound nature, known as combined stammering and stuttering. Here, also, their malady would yield readily to proper methods of treatment, but instead of giving it the attention so badly needed, they allow it to pass into a severe case of Spasmodic Stammering, and from this into the most chronic stage of that trouble. The malady becomes rooted in the muscular system. The nervous strain and continued fear tear down all semblance of mental control and in time the sufferer is in a condition that is hopeless indeed, a condition where he is subject for the pity and the sympathy of every one who stammers, and yet a condition brought on purely by his own neglect and wilfulness.

I recall the case of a father who brought his boy of 16 to see me some years ago. At that time, the boy represented one of the worst cases of stammering I ever saw. He could scarcely speak at all. He made awful contortions of the face and body when attempting to speak. When he succeeded in uttering sounds, these resembled the deep bark of a dog. These sounds were totally unintelligible, save upon rare occasions, when he would be able to speak clearly enough to make himself understood. I gave the boy the most searching personal diagnosis and very carefully inspected his condition both mental and physical, after which I was convinced that he could be cured, with time and persistent work. The father was given the result of my findings and told of the boy's condition. He decided to take the boy home, talk the matter over and place him under my care the next week. Ten days later he wrote me saying that the boy had secured a job in a garage at $6 a week and could not think about being cured of stammering at that time.

Two and a half years later--the boy was nearing twenty--I saw him again, and even after all my experience in meeting stammerers, could hardly believe that stammering could bring about such a terrible condition as this boy was in at that time. His mental faculties were entirely shattered. His concentration was gone. This poor boy was merely a blubbering, stumbling idiot, a sight to move the stoutest heart, a living example of the result of carelessness and parental neglect. Needless to say, I would not consider his treatment in such a condition. There was no longer any foundation to build on--no longer the slightest chance for benefiting the boy in the least.

THE WILFULLY DISOBEDIENT CASES: Taking up the fourth class of incurables, those who refuse to obey instructions--I can only say that such as these are not deserving of a cure. They are not sincere, they are not willing to hold themselves to the simplest program no matter how great might be the resultant good. They spend their own money or the money of their parents foolishly, get no results and disgust the instructor who spends his or her efforts in trying to bring about a cure, against obstacles that no one can overcome, viz.: unwillingness to do as told. The old saying that "You can lead a horse to water, but you can't make him drink" applies most forcefully to the case of the wilfully disobedient stammerer. You can instruct this individual in the methods to bring about a cure, but you can't make him follow them.

I well remember one case in point. A young man of 20 years came to me apparently with every desire in the world to be cured of stammering. The first day he followed instructions with great care, seemed to take a wonderful interest in his work and at the end of the day expressed to me his pleasure in finding himself improved even with one day's work. By the third day, the novelty had worn off and his "smart-aleck" tendencies began to come to the surface. He was impertinent. He was impudent. He was rude. He failed to come to his work promptly in the morning, was late at meals, stayed out at night beyond the time limit set by the dormitory rules and persisted in doing everything in an irregular and wilfully disobedient manner.

I was not inclined to dismiss him because of his misconduct, because it was evident that here was a boy of more than ordinary native intelligence, a fine-looking chap with untold opportunities ahead of him, if he were cured of stammering. So I put up with his misdeeds for many days, until one morning I decided that either he must come to time or return to his home--and he elected to take the latter course.

In looking up this boy's record later on, it was found that he was incorrigible, that his parents had never been successful in controlling him at any time and that he had been expelled from school twice.

There is no need for me to say that this boy was afflicted with something even worse than stammering--something that science was not able to help--i. e., a lack of sense. His case was incurable, just as much so as if an inch of his tongue had been sheared off. With such stammerers as this I have neither patience nor sympathy. They have no respect or consideration for others and are consequently entitled to none themselves.

THE CHRONIC DISSIPATOR: The fifth type of incurable might be called the "chronic dissipator" and his stammering is hopelessly incurable just as far as his habits are incurable. The person who persists in undermining his mental and physical being with dissipation and who, when he knows the results of his doings, will not cease, cannot hope to be cured of stammering. Cases such as these I do not attempt to treat. They are neither wanted nor accepted.

I recall the case of a man of 32, a big, stalwart fellow, who came to me about two years ago with a very severe case of combined stammering and stuttering. He made his plans to place himself under my care but before getting back, fell a victim to his inordinate appetite for drink and was laid up for a week. His wife wrote me the circumstances, told me it had been going on for nine years and that all efforts to eradicate the appetite had failed. I immediately advised her that I considered his case incurable and could not accept him for treatment. In such cases, a cure is built upon too shallow and uncertain a foundation to offer any hope of being permanent.

BELOW NORMAL INTELLIGENCE: There is another incurable case which must be included if we are to complete this list of the incurable forms of speech impediments. That is the case of the stammerer who is of below normal intelligence. These cases are very rare and I do not recall but four instances where a case has been diagnosed as incurable on account of the lack of intelligence. This is a direct refutation of the statement that stammerers are naturally below normal in mental ability. Out of more than twenty-six years' experience in meeting stammerers by the thousands, I can say most emphatically that stammerers as a class ARE NOT NATURALLY BELOW NORMAL INTELLIGENCE OR MENTAL POWER, SAVE AS THEIR TROUBLE MAY HAVE AFFECTED THEIR CONCENTRATION OR WILL-POWER.

THE LACKADAISICAL: The last and largest class of incurable cases of stammering are those who will not make the effort to be cured. These are the spineless, the unsure, the cowards, who are afraid to try anything for fear it will not be successful.

They are usually afflicted with a malady worse than stammering or stuttering--"indecision"--a malady for which science has found no remedy. Knowing the dire results of continued stammering, still they stammer. Reason fails to move them to the necessary effort. Common sense makes no appeal. Well, indeed, in such cases, may we paraphrase the words of Dr. Russell H. Conwell and say:

"There is nothing in the world that can prevent you from being cured of stammering but YOURSELF. Neither heredity, environment or any of the obstacles superimposed by man can keep you from marching straight through to a cure if you are guided by a firm, driving determination and have health and normal intelligence."

These seven classes of incurable cases complete the list. And the number of such cases, all taken together, is so small as to be almost out of consideration. For, out of a thousand cases of stuttering and stammering examined, I find but 2 per cent. with organic defects or of an incurable nature. In other words, 98 per cent. can be completely and permanently cured.

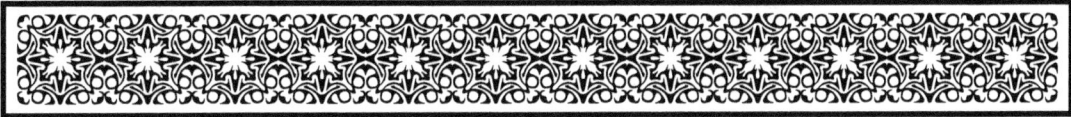

CHAPTER IV
CAN STAMMERING BE CURED BY MAIL?

In the years past there have been attempts from time to time to induce the stammerer to seek a cure for his impediment in mail order treatments. As has already been told, I was the victim of one of these so-called "correspondence-cures" and know something about them from personal experience.

In the first place, the sufferer usually takes up with the mail order specialist because this man retails his "profound" knowledge at a low rate, a rate so low that even a single thought on the subject would convince anyone that his money was buying a few sheets of paper but no professional knowledge or experience.

The very best correspondence course I have ever known anything about was not as good as a number of books on elocution that are available in any good library. Usually these courses are written by some charlatan who is in business as a mail-order-man selling trinkets and stammering cures or running a general correspondence school, teaching not only how to cure stammering by correspondence but giving courses in "Hair-Waving" and "How to Become a Detective." It is needless for me to say that such as these are in the business, not for the good of the stammerer nor even for the purpose of helping him, but simply for the money that can be extracted from the stammerer or stutterer.

THE DIFFERENCE: There are two main differences, however, between the books which the stammerer may read without cost and the correspondence course for which he pays out his good money--many dollars of it. The correspondence course has been written by a man who knew little or nothing of the subject, and who put out a course for stammerers only because he knew something of the number of stammerers in his territory and said to himself, "My, but I ought to be able to sell them a mail-order cure." Forthwith he sits down and writes a course--it isn't necessary to have anything in it at all. Often these men do not even take the trouble to consult reliable books on the subject. They do not profess to know anything about stammering or stuttering, their cause or their cure. They simply sit down and write--and when they have it written, they send it to the printer, have it printed and then split these printed sheets up into ten, or twenty, or fifty, or a hundred lessons--whatever their fancy may dictate, and begin to sell them. They have no thought of the results--results to them mean nothing save the number of courses that can be sold--and whether or not a single iota of good accrues to the stammerer from this expenditure of money is one of the things in which the correspondence school stammering specialist is not at all interested.

The most that can be expected from the very best mail course for the cure of stammering is that the subscriber will receive information worth as much as that which might be in a library book. He receives this in installments and for privilege of reading it piece-meal, pays from $50 to $100.

It is hopeless to try to cure stammering or stuttering by any method unless the instructor knows his business. And this knowledge comes not by chance but by long, hard study.

MAIL CURES A FAILURE: No stammerer should attempt to be cured by any correspondence method. When the decision has been made to have a speech defect removed, the sufferer should place himself under the care of a reputable institution, the past record of which entitles it to consideration. Correspondence cures are a waste of money, a waste of time and finally leave the stammerer with the firm-founded belief that his trouble is absolutely incurable, when, as a matter of fact, he may have a comparatively simple form of stuttering or stammering which could be quickly eradicated by the proper institutional treatment.

At no time should the stammerer resort to the use of any mechanical contrivance to aid him in speaking correctly. The cause of the trouble as previously explained, is inco-ordination. Mechanical contrivances to hold the tongue in a certain position, elevate the palate or for any other purpose may be positively harmful and should be strictly avoided--ALWAYS.

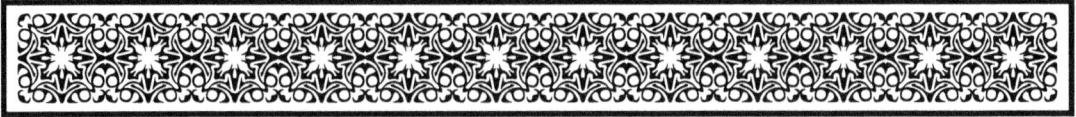

CHAPTER V
THE IMPORTANCE OF EXPERT DIAGNOSIS

A diagnosis is an examination or analysis to determine the identity of a disease and to reveal its cause and characteristics. A reputable medical man will not undertake the treatment of any malady without having first made a searching examination and a thorough diagnosis of the trouble.

In the case of the stammerer or stutterer, expert diagnosis is very important and should be undertaken only by a diagnostician who has had previous training and experience of sufficient duration to enable him to be classed as an expert on the subject. No stammerer or stutterer, however, should overlook the value of such diagnosis, for the reason that there are so many forms of speech disorders that it is totally impossible as well as unsafe for the sufferer himself to try to determine the exact nature of his trouble.

I recall the case of a certain young man who had depended upon his own knowledge to determine the identity of his speech defect and the nature of his trouble. When a boy, he had swallowed a small program pencil with a metal tip, injuring his vocal cords, so he said, and causing him to become a stammerer. An examination of his condition and a careful diagnosis of his case revealed the fact that his vocal organs were as normal as those of any person who had never stammered. The diagnosis also revealed the fact that his stammering was not originally caused by any organic defect or any injury to the vocal organs, but that, on the other hand, he had, in the first place, inherited a predisposition to stammer, his father and his grandfather both having been stammerers whose trouble had never been remedied. The diagnosis showed that the onset of the trouble immediately after swallowing the pencil was due chiefly to the nervous shock and fright caused by the accident, which, in conjunction, with the inherited predisposition toward stammering, was too much for the boy's mental control and he immediately developed into a stammerer. The young man had believed for many years that his defective utterance was totally incurable, that it was due to an organic defect which could not be remedied. The diagnosis quickly revealed, however, that a very different condition was responsible for his trouble and as a consequence, he found himself able to be cured where, without expert diagnosis, he had resigned himself to a life as a stammerer.

Another case which also shows the stammerer's inability to diagnose his own trouble accurately was that of a woman who persistently refused to allow her son to have his case diagnosed, because of her belief that he was incurable and that the diagnosis would be a waste of time and money.

After months of coaxing, however, he succeeded in getting her to consent and I gave him a thorough diagnosis and report on his condition. This mother had been unduly alarmed--the boy was still in a curable stage and in fact completed the necessary work in much less than the usual time. This is but another case that shows the loss which comes from not knowing the truth.

Written Report of Diagnosis Valuable: It is well to get a personal diagnosis of the case where possible, but if this cannot be done, a written history of the case, together with a statement of the symptoms and present condition, should enable the expert diagnostician of speech defects to make a thorough and reliable diagnosis of the trouble.

This diagnosis, to be of the most value to the stammerer or stutterer, should be made up in the form of a written report, so that the information may be in permanent form and so that the sufferer can study his own case in all its angles.

WHAT DIAGNOSIS SHOULD SHOW: First of all, of course, the diagnosis should identify and label your trouble. It should tell what form of speech defect is revealed by the symptoms; it should tell the cause of the trouble; the stage it is now in; should indicate whether or not there is any organic defect; should give information as to the possibilities of outgrowing the trouble; and, most important of all, should state whether or not the disorder is in a curable stage.

When it is remembered that nearly a dozen more or less common speech disorders can be named, almost in one breath, and that some of these disorders may pass through four or five successive stages, it will be seen that an expert diagnosis and report is almost a necessity to the stammerer or stutterer who would have reliable and authoritative information about his speech disorder.

The stammerer or stutterer who voluntarily remains in the dark, who is satisfied with gross ignorance of his trouble, is surely not on the road to freedom of speech.

The most able man cannot decide correctly without the facts. To decide in the absence of information is guesswork--and guesswork is a poor method of deciding what to do--in the case of the stammerer as in every other case.

Therefore, it behooves the stammerer to become enlightened to as great an extent as possible, to banish ignorance of his trouble and replace it with facts and sound knowledge.

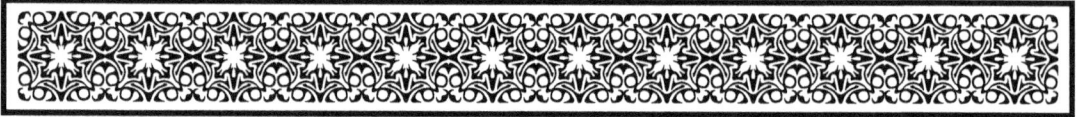

CHAPTER VI
THE SECRET OF CURING STUTTERING AND STAMMERING

If the reader has followed this work carefully up to this point, he is now informed on the causes of stuttering and stammering, on their characteristic tendencies and their peculiarities. We are now ready to ask, "What are the correct methods for the cure of stuttering and stammering?" and to answer that question authoritatively.

As to the successful mode of procedure in determining the proper methods for the cure of stuttering and stammering, I know of no suggestion better than that offered by Alexander Melville Bell, who says:

"The rational, as it is experimentally the successful method of procedure, is first to study the standard of correct articulation (NOT the varieties of imperfect utterance) and then not to go from one extreme to another, but at every step to compare the defective with the perfect mode of speech and so infallibly to ascertain the amount, the kind and the source of the error."

We have already done that: We have located the cause of the trouble. We not only know that stammering is caused by a lack of co-ordination between the brain and the muscles of speech, but we know the things which may bring about the lack of co-ordination. Now, how to cure? Simply remove the cause. Re-establish normal co- ordination between the brain and the muscles of speech. Restore normal brain control over the speech organs. Make these organs respond freely, naturally and promptly to the brain messages.

That sounds simple. But if it is as simple as it sounds, why is it that so many in the past have failed to cure stammering and stuttering? Why have so many so-called methods of cure passed into the discard? The answer is, they were based on the wrong foundation. They struck at the effects and not at the cause of the trouble. And as a result, the methods failed.

These so-called methods have aimed at many different effects. One method, for instance, had as its theory that if you could cure the nervousness, the stammering would magically disappear. The unfortunate sufferer was doped with vile-tasting bitters and nerve medicines, so-called, in the hope that his nervous system would respond to treatment. But the nerves could not be quieted and the nervous system built up until the cause of the nervousness--which was stammering--was removed.

There was a time, too, and it has not been so long ago, when the craze was on for using surgery as a cure-all for stammering. Terrible butchery was performed in the name of surgery--the patient's tongue sometimes being slitted or notched, and other foolish and cruel subterfuges improvised in an effort to cure the stammering. Needless to say, there was no cure found in such methods. There is no chance of curing a mental defect by slitting the tongue and the absurdities of that "butchering period" which have now passed away, are numbered among the mistakes of those who committed them.

A lack of thoroughness marked the later attempts to cure stammering. One method was based, for instance, solely upon correct breathing. There is no doubt that correct breathing is very vital both to the stammerer and the non-stammerer, if they are to speak fluently and well. But breath-control does not even begin to solve the problem of curing stammering. It is but an element, and a small element, in the proper articulation of words. And however well this plan of breath-control might have succeeded, it could never have succeeded in really curing stuttering and stammering.

Most of these ill-advised efforts and half-baked methods sprang up, not as a result of sound knowledge but rather as a result of the lack of it. In fact, looking back at the manner in which the stammerer was treated for stammering under these methods, we can see now that nothing but the most profound ignorance of the fundamental principles underlying the art of speaking could have made it possible for these misguided instructors to pass out as science the jargon and hodge-podge which they did try to pass off as scientific knowledge. The absurdities propounded in the name of stammering cures were too numerous even to enumerate in this volume.

SPEECH PRINCIPLES FUNDAMENTAL: Back of every spoken word, whether that word be French, English, Italian, or any other language, are the unchangeable principles of speech. These principles of speech are fundamental. They do not change basically nor do they vary in the individual. When you speak correctly, you do so as a result of following the correct principles of speech. I speak correctly by the same method as you. And when you speak incorrectly, or when you stutter or stammer, you do so because you have violated one or more of these fundamental principles. Any other person who stammers or stutters as you do, violates the same principles and requires the same method of correction as yourself. The severity of your case depends upon how many of the principles of speech you violate. A diagnosis will determine this--and therefore what is necessary to be done to bring about perfect speech. The number of speech violations to be corrected will also determine to a certain extent the time required for correction.

SPEECH DEFINED: Speech, in all the diversities of tongues and dialects, consists of but a small number of articulated elementary sounds. These are produced by the agency of the lungs, the larynx, and the mouth. The lungs supply air to the larynx, which modifies the stream into whisper or voice; and this air is then moulded by the plastic oral organs into syllables which singly or in accentual combinations constitute words.

As explained in the Chapter on Causes, all of the physical organs which have to do with the production of speech and all of the brain centers whose duty it is to control the actions of these various organs, must operate in harmony, or, in other words, must coordinate, if we are to have perfect speech. Co-ordination implies perfect mental control of physical actions. And this in turn means perfect obedience of the physical organs of speech to the brain messages that are received.

The cure of stammering and stuttering requires a great deal of care based, of course, upon the correct scientific knowledge in the first place.

In attempting to cure stammering, there has been too much teaching by rigid rules and not enough teaching by principles. There are very few hard-and-fast rules that can be followed with success by every stutterer or stammerer. No set of rules can be laid down as a standard for every one to follow, for no two persons stammer exactly alike any more than two persons look exactly alike.

The only safe rule of all the rules is that which says, "Cleave closely to the principles, let the rules fall where they may." The only successful method is that which, being first based upon the right principle, is followed out with intelligence by the stammerer and administered with wisdom by the instructor to fit the needs and requirements of the individual case.

METHODS NECESSARILY THREE-FOLD: The cure of stammering and stuttering can be wrought only by a method that is three-fold-that attacks all of the un-normal conditions of the stammerer simultaneously and eradicates them in unison.

It would be of little avail, for instance, to build up perfect breath control, and leave the stammerer in a mental state where he was continually harassed by a fear of failure, by a continual self-consciousness and irritated by a deep-seated nervousness.

And it would be of just as little use to try to remove that self- consciousness, fear of failure and nervousness without removing the cause of the stammering.

In other words, when the successful method of curing stammering is spoken of as being threefold in purpose, it is meant that this method must build up the physical being, must achieve perfect mental equilibrium and must link up the physical with the mental in perfect harmony.

A permanent cure can rest on no other foundation than perfect restoration to a truly normal mental and physical condition. When this has been accomplished and when the synchronization of brain and speech organs has been brought about, the muscles of speech do not hesitate in responding to a brain message for the utterance of a word. There is no longer any sticking, any loose or hurried repetition. In other words, perfect speech now comes as a logical consequence.

SPEECH SPECIALIST SHOULD HAVE STAMMERED: It is very important that the speech expert who would promulgate a method for the eradication of stammering should have, at one time or another, stammered himself.

It is a well-known fact that the imagination cannot conjure up an image of something that has never been experienced. If you had been born blind, you would have no mental picture of any color, no matter how much you might have heard about it. Still your imagination might be a most prolific one. The utmost feat of the human imagination is to combine mental pictures to form still other images which are impossible or absurd or which in their entirety have not been experienced. In other words, new combinations of images are possible, but an entirely new or basic picture is beyond the power of the imagination to create.

So, with the specialist who would cure stuttering and stammering. It is impossible for the man who has never stammered or stuttered to know the fear that grips the sufferer when he thinks of speaking. It is impossible for one who has never stammered to imagine what this fear is like or to know the feeling that accompanies it.

For that reason, it is important that the man who attempts to eradicate speech defects should have been afflicted himself in order that his experience may have been acquired first-hand--that the suffering may have been felt and all of the conditions and situations of the stammerer may be as familiar to him as to his student.

Value of Moral Influence in the Cure of Stammering: In speaking of the necessity for good health, both physical and mental, before the eradication of stammering can take place, we must not overlook a few words about one particular type of derelict--the will-less or sometimes wilful individual who persists in indulging in dissipation of every kind, the individual who, with cocksure attitude and haughty sneer, laughs in the face of experience and insists that "it will not bother him." To such as these, no hope can be held out. Such tactics leave both body and mind in a condition that does not permit of up-building. There is little foundation for any effort and with the passing of each day, there is a tearing-out of bodily and mental vigor that makes all effort useless.

But in the average individual, physical rebuilding is a process of but a few weeks. The mental rehabilitation can usually be accomplished in an equally short period of time and when these things have been brought about, perfect speech soon follows if the correct methods are applied.

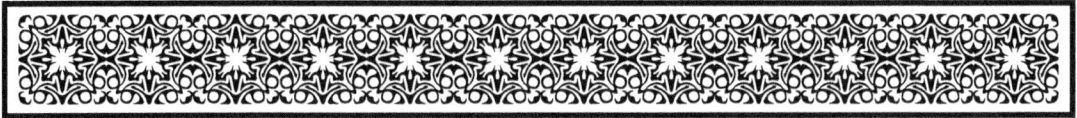

CHAPTER VII
THE BOGUE UNIT METHOD DESCRIBED

At the time a stammerer or stutterer first places himself under my care and before any attempt is made to apply the treatment, he is given a very thorough and searching examination for the purpose of learning the exact nature of his difficulty. It must be remembered that no two cases of stammering or stuttering are exactly alike and that no two cases require exactly the same method of treatment, although the same basic principles apply to all.

Even if the stammerer's case has been previously diagnosed by me, it is necessary to compare and verify the symptoms as previously exhibited with those existing at the time of his beginning treatment, in order to learn, first of all, whether his malady has more recently progressed into a further and more serious stage.

The Bogue Test: If the usual entrance examination does not bring out all of the essential facts regarding the case, the stammerer is then put through the Bogue Test--an original system of diagnosis which I perfected some years ago--by means of which the peculiarities of the trouble are brought out, the NORMAL, the SUB-NORMAL and the ABNORMAL condition of the disorder is gauged and the most minute details of the trouble are disclosed. This Bogue Test covers the case from every possible angle. It lays bare the exact physical, mental and nervous condition of the stammerer or stutterer, enables me to determine the original cause of the trouble and to follow its progress from the first up to the present time, almost as easily as if the student had been under my observation ever since he first noticed his defect of speech.

I recall the case of a boy who came to me at one time for a personal diagnosis of his case. I examined him carefully, put him through a number of tests and diagnosed his case, which proved to be in the second stage and of no more than ordinary severity. He was unable to place himself under my care at that tune but returned to me about eight months later, apparently in no worse condition than before. Not being satisfied with the results of the examination, the complete test was applied, with the result that a condition of grave seriousness was discovered, marking the most pronounced form of his trouble--a form so far advanced as to make the case almost incurable. The situation was explained to the young man and he was told that it would take much longer than usual to bring about a cure in his case, although such a cure was yet possible. He expressed his willingness to spend as much time as was necessary in the cure and as a result, he was able within some weeks' time to talk without stuttering or stammering. The mental sluggishness which marked his conversation soon disappeared. He became alert and eager and when he left for home, he was a much different boy than when he came for treatment.

This is but one of hundreds of examples showing the need for expert diagnosis and for careful analysis of the condition of the stammerer even if a previous diagnosis has been made within a few months.

In practically all cases of stammering, particularly those of a progressive character, the condition is naturally changeable and common prudence calls for caution in accepting antedated facts as an indication of the present condition.

In every case, the examination enables me to gauge the severity of the case so accurately that the student's course can be outlined, designating the exact Plan-of-Attack to be used in:

1--Tearing out the improper methods of speech production
2--Replacing those incorrect methods with the correct natural
  methods
3--Re-establishing normal co-ordination between the brain and
  the muscles of speech.

The Method at Work: When the preliminary Examination and Tests have been completed and the student's course outlined, the actual working of the Bogue Unit Method then begins. This does not involve the practice of any "ism" or "ology," nor does it require the use of medicines, drugs, surgery, hypnotism or the "laying-on-of-hands," but by scientific and natural methods, begins the first step of the work, viz.: Tearing out the improper methods of speech production.

At every step in the application of the method, the principles which underlie and govern perfect articulation, serve as the foundation of the instruction. As has been so often stated in this book, these principles of speech never change. They apply to all persons alike, and all who talk normally apply these principles in the same manner. Those who stammer violate them, so that in correcting defective speech it is only logical that we should first remove the defective procedure and then institute the correct procedure in its place.

The Bogue Unit Method is three-fold in action. From this it takes the name "Unit Method." The first Unit of Treatment has for its purpose the building up of physical efficiency. "The first requisite is to be a good animal," says Herbert Spencer. This is certainly true of the stammerer, for in his case, normal health is a valuable aid during the time of treatment. Consequently, the first step is to build up the physical organs and be sure that these are functioning properly.

The second Unit of Treatment restores the mental equilibrium, stabilizes the mental activities and places them under perfect control. The inability of the mind to control the organs of speech has led to a condition which might be described as a "flabbiness of the mental muscles" which necessitates that the mental condition be altered and improved so that the mind can once more possess the capacity for properly controlling the organs of speech.

The third Unit of Treatment synchronizes and harmonizes mental and physical actions and re-establishes normal co-ordination between the brain and the muscles of speech, which completes the work necessary to bring about a cure. After both physical and mental conditions have been made normal, it merely remains to link up these two properly-working forces, co-ordinate their activities and firmly inhabitate the correct principles of control, after which it can be said that a complete cure is permanently effected.

Daily Record of Progress: Beginning with the first day, a complete report in writing is made of the progress. Each point on which the student makes progress is noted. If proper advancement is not made on any particular point, special effort is put forth to bring that point up to the standard which has been set. This makes it possible for the instructor to give individual attention to each student, something which is absolutely essential in many cases. In other words, it will not do to start the student off and let him work out his own salvation. The instructor must be constantly at hand, giving advice, correcting faulty articulation and constantly aiding the stammerer in a hundred ways to route the malady.

After having been under treatment for seven days, the student is subjected to his first treatment test. After passing this examination satisfactorily, the student is assigned additional work from another angle. Some students require as much as ten days to complete the work necessary to pass this first test--in fact, it might also be said that this test will determine the speed with which the student is to progress. From this time until the completion of the course, additional tests are given at various intervals, according to the needs of the case, until the Final Cure Test proves that the malady has been eradicated.

Conscious of the Improvement: The stammerer is profoundly conscious of a distinct change for the better by the end of the very first day under treatment. In other words, there is an immediate and noticeable improvement, not only in his nervous condition, but also in his physical and mental state as well.

Before the student passes from under the treatment, he is thoroughly aware of the benefits which the work has brought about. For, after he has met every progress test and has been examined on every phase and every principle of speech, he passes to a rigid Final Test. In this test, more than ever before, he finds the results of his efforts. He discovers that he can use his speech in any way that he desires--in any way that it will be necessary for him to use it in his future life. He finds himself able to produce any sound--labial, dental, lingual, nasal or palatal or any combination of these sounds in any language. He finds every word now is an easy word, articulation is under perfect control and the formation of voice a process involving no apparent mental effort or physical contortions.

A young woman of 20 years was placed under my care by her mother. She stammered very badly and at the time when her condition was at its worst, found it almost impossible to make herself understood by any means. After five weeks of careful instruction, this young woman had no difficulty whatever in speaking, there was no "piling up of thoughts," as she expressed her former condition, and her articulation was excellent. A few days after she returned home, she wrote as follows: "I have been talking ever since I came home and have had no trouble whatever. I just love to talk and I believe I have said more in the last five days than in the whole last five years."

Additional Results: The Bogue Unit Method of Cure when earnestly followed out by the student, does much more than eradicate the impediment of speech. It increases the weight of the below-the- average student, stops all spasmodic or convulsive efforts of face, arms and limbs and increases by several inches what was formerly a flat and poorly developed chest.

A very bad case who came to me for treatment several years ago was a young man of 26. He not only stuttered but stammered very badly. He placed himself under my guidance for a period of a little more than six weeks. At the end of that time he found no difficulty in talking nor were there any spasmodic movements of the facial muscles, as before. In reporting some time later, he said:

"When I left I tipped the scales at 20 pounds heavier than when I went to you. My folks are certainly pleased to hear me talk without the straining and strangling exertion I had before in trying to force my words out. Now they flow out nice and easy."

Many children, both boys and girls, are under developed. This may have resulted from several causes, but it is frequently traceable to the stammering or stuttering as an indirect cause. The Bogue Unit Method takes these children in a poor physical condition and while eradicating the defect of speech, brings about a healthy physical development. An Ohio woman reported excellent results in a letter which said:

"I am glad to inform you that my son Allan since taking the treatment in June last, has not to my knowledge, stammered once, for which we are all very grateful to the Bogue Method. I also wish to say that his physical condition is much improved and he has increased in weight about ten pounds."

Regardless of the age of the student, there is an increased vitality flowing through the entire body, the powers of endurance are greatly increased and the health built up from every stand- point. One man sent in an enthusiastic report in these words:

"I am fine and healthy; the people down here say I don't look like the same person. I gained 17 pounds while I was out there. I am talking fine. My mother says I talk them nearly to death. I talk them all to bed at night, so they put out the light on me so I will go to bed and hush. I went down town Saturday night and the boys were sure glad to hear me talk without stammering."

Even THIS physical improvement is not unusual.

Another man reports the change brought about in his condition as follows:

"Just about two years ago I was one of the worst stammerers I know that ever was; it was simply awful. I could not speak a word without the most terrible stammering you ever heard. My parents were heartbroken over my condition, which grew worse all the time. I did not grow and develop like my brothers. My shoulders were stooped, my chest sunken--in fact, I was in a terrible condition. After staying with you for six weeks I came home and every one who knew me when I left was simply astonished at the improvement, not in my speech alone, but in my physical condition also. Am stronger and well now and I say it is a comfort to be able to talk like other boys."

This case is not an unusual one, however, for it is frequently found that the stammering child grows into a physically deficient man as a result of his speech impediment.

Concomitant with these physical betterments comes a changed mental attitude, whereby the former pessimistic outlook has been changed to an optimistic view of life. The former abnormal timidity of the student has been replaced by a perfect confidence; the old unreasoning fear-of-failure is transformed into a feeling of supreme self-reliance; and the depressed, care-worn expression which may once have marked the stammerer's countenance has given place to that of cheerfulness.

The weak and vacillating will now manifests itself as a dominant, masterful power-of-will and the stagnant mentality of the stammerer has now given place to a vigorous, forceful, creative mental power. The mind-wandering or lack of ability to concentrate is gone and in its place is an intense and well controlled power- of-concentration. In addition to this, the nervousness which marked the every movement of the stammerer has disappeared and the self-consciousness which made life a misery is replaced by a calm self-control, resulting in an entire self-forgetfulness, perfect poise and a feeling of self-possession.

These benefits accrue gradually as the course progresses, but when, upon the completion of the course, perfect speech is finally restored, the results are fully evident and entirely permanent. Their permanency is the crowning result of the proper methods-- methods which eradicate the trouble at its source--treat and remove the cause instead of treating the effect.

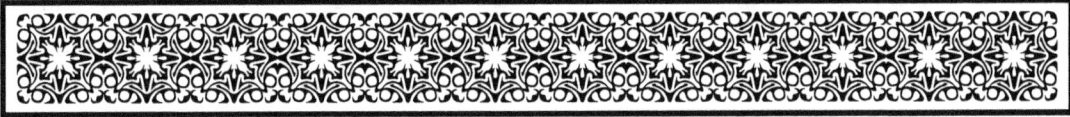

CHAPTER VIII
SOME CASES I HAVE MET

During the last twenty-eight years, I have personally met more than 22,000 stammerers, diagnosed 97,000 cases by mail and corresponded with more than 210,000 people who stammer or stutter. In this time, it is only natural that I should have come in contact with almost every conceivable type of stammering in practically every form.

I am going to describe a few of these cases in this chapter, give their history and description very briefly, follow out the course of the trouble when unchecked and indicate the circumstances of cure when the stammerer has placed himself for treatment.

I shall make no attempt to discuss all types of speech disorders nor even all of the forms of any one type, but rather to take up those cases which can be regarded as most common and which are typical of the disorders of the largest number of stammerers and stutterers. Since a whole volume could easily be filled with descriptions of cases, it is evident that those discussed here must be but briefly described.

(The case numbers in the following pages refer to specific cases, but not to the order of their treatment, since the classification is a decimal system used to indicate type, duration, stage, etc.)

Case No. 65.435--This was a boy of 8, brought to me by his mother after he had experienced untold trouble in school. The boy complained of a pain in his head when making an effort to talk or after having spoken under the strain for some minutes. I found the spasmodic contractions accompanying his trouble to be very pronounced for a boy so young in years and upon making the examination, was not surprised to find his to be a case of Combined Stammering and Stuttering. There was no indication of Thought-Lapse, but there was a condition that could easily have been mistaken for it--viz.: a woeful lack of confidence in his own ability to speak, which in this boy's case was due to the fact that he had stuttered almost since his first word and had rarely spoken words correctly. As has been previously explained, every child learns to speak by imitation and his confidence in his speaking-ability must be gained by constant reassurance from some source that he is speaking correctly. Early in life this boy had found that he was NOT speaking correctly and at that moment began to feel the lack of confidence which had been growing upon him daily. Although in the midst of his school work, arrangements were easily made to remove him from class and place him for treatment. Notwithstanding the fact that his trouble was unusually severe for a boy of that age, seven weeks at the Institute saw him made into a new boy, his confidence regained, his speech under perfect control and his physical condition greatly improved. He returned to school, where his unusual proficiency enlisted the aid and co- operation of his teachers to such an extent that he was able to finish the semester with his class.

Case No. 7.232--This was another boy of early school age, whose case is described here because of the contrast of the one just mentioned. The present case was that of a boy soon to be 10 years old. He had stammered, not since his first word, but only since he had been allowed to play with two children, twins, who lived in the neighborhood, and both of whom had stuttered since their first attempts to speak. While I never examined the twins, it seems from what I learned of them, that the predisposition to stammer was an inherited one, both the father and grandfather having been inveterate stammerers. Be that as it may, their defective enunciation, practiced in the presence of the boy whose case I am describing, caused the boy himself to acquire a habit of imperfect enunciation which took the form of simple stuttering and which all the home efforts of his mother and father had failed to eradicate. At the time he was brought to me, I gave him the usual examination, traced his trouble back to its original cause-- Unconscious Imitation diagnosed his case as one of Simple Stuttering and recommended the procedure to be followed. This boy left my care after three weeks and experienced no further difficulty to this day, although he is now 24 years old and engaged in work that necessitates his making impromptu speeches almost every day. Here was a case of Simple Stuttering, taken at the right time, which yielded almost magically to the treatment, but had it been allowed to run on, would have progressed into the Advanced Stage of

Stuttering and later, in all probability, into an extremely severe case of Combined Stammering and Stuttering.

Case No. 986.523--This was the case of a Polish boy who found it almost impossible to begin a word or a sentence. In describing his case to me, he finally managed to say, "Before I utter a word it takes me a long time and after I utter the word, I become red in the face and so excited that I don't know where I am, or what I am doing!" I found this boy to be extremely high-strung and of a nervous temperament, easily excited. He was of an emotional type, was more-than-ordinarily sensitive about his trouble and brooded over it constantly, having long fits of deep melancholia that were a constant source of worry to his parents. He was furthermore at a critical age, from the standpoint of his speech development, just approaching 16. Although naturally of an agreeable disposition, his trouble had made him irritable and often sullen. He wore an air of dejection almost constantly. It was evident to me immediately upon examination that his trouble had had a grave effect upon his mind and that it would in time (and not so long a time, either) have a deep and permanent effect that no amount of effort could eradicate.

It would be naturally expected that his symptoms would indicate Thought-Stammering, but this is not true. Instead I found his to be a bad case of Spasmodic Stammering, in which the convulsive action took place immediately upon an effort to speak and which resulted, therefore, in the inability to express a sound--the "sticking" tendency so common to stammering and particularly to this type.

While the worry over his stammering had left him in a mental state that made him impotent so far as normal mental accomplishments were concerned, still the removal of his stammering by the eradication of the cause would, I felt, entirely relieve the condition of mental flurry and stop the nervousness.

The case was so urgent that the boy's parents decided to place him for treatment immediately. The results were so gratifying as to be almost unbelievable. By the end of the first day's work, the boy's whole mental attitude was changed. His outlook on life was different. He felt the thrill of conquering his difficulty and before many days, he was working like a Trojan to make his cure complete and permanent. At my suggestion, he remained with me for seven weeks, at the end of which time he went back East, entirely changed in every particular. He was smiling now, where before he seemed to have forgotten how to smile. He was full of life, enthusiasm and ambition--no one who had seen him the day he first came here, could realize that this was the same boy that entered a few weeks before with the desire-to-live almost extinct. There are hundreds of cases riot far different from this--I have cited the case of this Polish boy to show what a complete transformation is made in the mental state by a few weeks' work along the right lines.

Case No. 87.522--Here was a case of a type that is very, very common. It was that of a girl, 17 years of age, from a good family, well-educated and having all the marks of careful training in a home of refinement. The most marked characteristic of her case was the tendency to recur. In other words, she was an Intermittent Stammerer, who had believed (as had her parents) that the tendency to get better was an indication that she would soon outgrow the trouble. "If Marie still stammers by the time she is 18--" this had come to be almost a household word, for if she stammered at that time, it was the intention of her parents (so they said) to have the girl placed under treatment. As was to be expected, she continued to stammer and continued to get steadily worse, although the tendency to be better and worse by turns was maintained throughout the years. The periods of improvement were eagerly seized by her parents, year after year, as indications of out-growing, while the periods of relapse were seldom spoken of and usually ignored. It was another case of the old saying that: "We like to think that the thing will happen which we want to happen," and since they wanted the daughter to outgrow her trouble, they insisted in believing, despite their own unexpressed fears, that the daughter would "eventually get over it!"

She did not get over it, however, and the critical age of 16 brought on a condition so severe that her parents became alarmed about her and sought advice as to what should be done.

An examination of her case brought out the fact that she had probably inherited a predisposition to stammer, but that the immediate cause of the trouble had been fright, caused by a nurse who had tried to discipline the girl when small, by telling her that the "bogey-man" would get her if she didn't do certain things as told. This disciplining by means of fear is never a safe procedure and in this case had been carried to extremes on many occasions, finally resulting in the child becoming a stammerer.

She had a case of Genuine Stammering in its second stage and, according to her own statement at the time the examination was made, had become much worse in the last two years. At age 15 it seems that everyone felt secure in the belief that her trouble would pass away, but at age 17, the condition became critical, the disorder having previously passed into the second stage.

Two and a half weeks worked a wonderful improvement in the girl's condition, at the end of which time she was compelled to return to her home on account of a death in the family. She remained at home for almost a month, after which she returned to me to complete the cure. Even under such an unusual and unfavorable circumstance as this, she remained with me the last time only four weeks, and has, according to her report, never stammered since, nor has she been oppressed by the overpowering sense of fear that formerly seized her when she thought of trying to talk.

Case No. 84.563--This case first came to my attention over ten years ago, when I was called upon to make a diagnosis. This showed the trouble to be a case of Combined Stammering and Stuttering, originally caused, it seemed, from having associated with an old man who was janitor in a wood-working plant belonging to the father of the boy whose case I am describing. The janitor had stammered ever since anyone about the place had known him and probably all of his life. In his early days, with his youth to carry him on, he had tried to hold down several jobs of consequence, but with varying success, dropping down the ladder rung by rung until he reached the place of janitor. The boy in question, having associated with the old man, early acquired the habit of mocking his defective speech, with the result that he himself soon began to stutter, which later turned into a combined form of disorder known as Combined Stammering and Stuttering.

He came to me at the time he was 28, having found it necessary to go to work on his own account, upon the failure of his father's business. I explained to him that his was a case of Combined Stammering and Stuttering, outlined to him the probable course of his trouble and what he might reasonably expect if he allowed it to continue. Having been married only a short time and being rather reluctant to leave home for the length of time necessary to take the course, he decided to postpone treatment until some later date. I heard nothing more from him for almost three years, when he walked in one day, looking like a shadow of his former self. There were dark rings around his eyes, his gaze was shifty and I could hardly believe that this was the young fellow who had seen me three years ago. Nevertheless it was the same man, with a story that pointed out the danger of postponement. His trouble had become steadily worse, he said, until it had ruined his control over himself. He had become nervous, irritable and cross, without meaning to be so, had lost one good position after another and finally, as a climax to a long string of misfortunes, his wife had left him. declaring that she would not put up with him in such a condition.

A second examination revealed the fact that his stammering had progressed so rapidly since he had last talked with me, that it was now perilously near the stage known as Thought Lapse. His control was not entirely shattered, however, and he was accepted for treatment. It was something over two months before he was back in shape again, but those two months did a wonderful thing for him, for it put him in first-class physical condition, removed all traces of his impediment and restored the mental equilibrium which had been so long endangered. Later, as a result of his restoration to perfect speech, his family differences were adjusted, and at the last reports, he was making splendid headway in a business of his own. Such is the power of stammering to destroy--even home and happiness itself--and such the power of perfect speech to build up again.

Case No. 465.722--This was the case of a man born in Ireland, who came to this country as a boy, and the original cause of whose trouble was a blow over the head in a street fight soon after landing in America.

When he came to me, he was 52 years of age and not only had one of the most severe cases of Spasmodic Stammering I have ever seen, but was in the first stages of Thought Lapse. He was practically speechless all of the time and his trouble instead of manifesting an Intermittent Tendency as it had formerly done, was now constant, indicating that he was in the chronic stage of his difficulty. Aside from his Spasmodic Stammering, he seemed unable to think of the things which he wished to say. In other words, his trouble had been affecting him so long that he had lost the power to recall and control the mental images necessary to the formation of words.

I not only gave him the usual examination but applied the special Bogue test, both of which convinced me that his case was far into the incurable stage. There was little or nothing I could do for him at that late date and so I told him. He acted as if dazed for a few moments, and when the full force of the truth dawned upon him, it was as if a cord had snapped and broken. Hope was gone. He was an incurable--and knew it now, only too well. And as he turned and left me, I knew from the droop of the shoulders and the hang of the head, that life meant but little to him now. He was merely waiting--waiting for the last page to be written and his book of despair to be closed.

Case No. 34.444--This young woman was very talented, had a beautiful singing voice and could not understand why she was unable to speak fluently when she could sing so well. The cause of her trouble was distinctly mental and did not lie in any defective formation of the vocal organs but rather in a lack of co- ordination between the brain and the muscles of speech. In her case, the speech disorder had not materially affected her health, although she admitted it had impaired her power of will and her ability to concentrate. Six weeks put her in good condition and gave her the opportunity to use her beautiful voice to excellent advantage in speaking as well as in singing--much to her satisfaction.

Case No. 667.788--This man came to me for assistance and relief from a severe case of Combined Stammering and Stuttering. He shook like a leaf when he talked, was very nervous, and could hardly sit still. His speech was marked by loose and hurried repetitions of syllables and words, alternating with a slow and seemingly dazed repetition of words, as though he did not know what he was saying.

In a few moments, I learned that he was a habitual alcoholic, that he was acquainted with the Delirium Tremens and that he frequently went upon sprees lasting a week, which left him a physical wreck. He had no backbone, there was no foundation to build on and his case was declined as incurable, not altogether from the condition of his speech, but because it is useless and hopeless to attempt treatment of the stammerer who is also a chronic dissipator.

Case No. 34.343--This was the case of a young man who came to me at the age of 17. He was one of the type that "seldom stammer." He explained this to me and told me that many of his friends were not aware of the fact that he stammered.

I gave him an examination and found his trouble to be a case of Combined Stammering and Stuttering in the second stage. He was of the Intermittent Type and at intervals his trouble became very bad, at which times he made it a point not to go out among his friends--one of the reasons which made it possible for him to say that his friends did not know of his speech trouble.

This young man came to me hoping that I would tell him that his trouble was not severe and that he would outgrow it in a few years. I was able to tell him that at the time his case was not an extremely bad one, but I knew that instead of being outgrown it would become ingrown, and I so told him.

But he decided to postpone action until some later date, feeling sure, despite what I had told him, that he would outgrow his stammering.

Four and a half years later, he came back. This time he did not say that his friends knew nothing of his trouble. He was in bad condition, his "seldom stammering," as he had called it, was chronic now and the painful expression on his face when he tried to talk was ample proof of the condition in which he had allowed himself to get. His trouble had passed into Genuine Stammering and was of a very severe nature. There was no thought of postponement in his mind at this time and he placed himself for treatment immediately. Eight weeks' time saw his work completed, with excellent results. His fear was gone, his confidence renewed and his health greatly improved, in addition to being able to talk fluently.

Case No. 66.788--Here was the case of a man of 30, a preacher, who found no difficulty in preaching to his congregation, from the pulpit, but whose trouble immediately got the best of him the moment he went down into the church and attempted to carry on a conversation individually. This became so embarrassing to him that he finally gave up the idea of passing through his congregation, but satisfied himself with standing at the door and greeting them as they passed out. This, too, he was later compelled to give up on account of his speech, although during none of this time did he have the slightest trouble in delivering his sermons.

His was a case of Genuine Stammering. The mental control when he was in the pulpit was almost normal. Talking to individuals, this control was quickly shattered. He placed himself for treatment after having secured a brother-pastor to fill his place for two months. He was a good student, obedient to instruction, concentrating on his work with a creditable energy. As a result, in five weeks' time, he found himself able to talk to anybody under any condition without the slightest sticking or fear. He could talk over the telephone and was master of himself under the cross-fire of conversation which in his previous state had bothered him so seriously.

Case No. 48.336--This is a case that represents a very common type of Combined Stammering and Stuttering, and a type that is not so quickly cured as might be imagined. This was a young man of 18, who not only stammered but stuttered. His speech disorder, however, was further complicated by a bad habit of prefixing a totally foreign word or sound to the word or sound which he found it difficult to pronounce. "B" was one of his hard sounds and in speaking the sentence: "We expect to leave Baltimore," he would say: "We expect to leave ah--ah--ah--Baltimore."

The fear of failure which caused him to acquire this habit of speaking, led his friends often to think that his mind wandered, although as a matter of fact, he was a very bright young fellow, without a single indication of Thought Lapse.

I diagnosed his case as Combined Stammering and Stuttering, and explained to him that he represented a type of stammering that might be called the "Prefix Stammerer" because of their habit of prefixing every hard sound with an easy word or an easy sound, even to the extent of losing the sense of the sentence--so great is the "Prefix Stammerer's" fear of failure.

He placed himself for treatment, and although his trouble was complicated by this prefixing habit, seven weeks put him in good shape. He forgot his fear of failure, found every word an easy word and every sound an easy sound. He learned to talk fluently again and returned to his home, both physically and mentally improved.

Case No. 98.656--This was the case of a rather arrogant young man from a good family, who was too proud to admit that he was a stammerer. Rather it should be said, he was too foolish to admit it. He was well-educated and with the store of words at his command, succeeded for some years in concealing the fact that he stammered. This he accomplished by the substitution of words. That is, words beginning with those letters that he could not utter were not used. If his sentence included such a word, he quickly substituted another word of somewhat similar meaning, but beginning with a letter that he could pronounce correctly. This substitution of words was so well done that for some time it was scarcely noticeable to the average listener. Often he found himself incorrectly understood, because of his inability to use the right word in the right place, but nevertheless he was successful in concealing his speech defect from many of his friends.

This case is of a type known as the "Synonym Stammerer" because synonyms are used to avoid stammering. The mental strain of trying always to substitute easy words for hard ones, was very great, however, and after a few years' practice, the strain began to tell on the young man. It affected his health and made him nervous and irritable.

It was at this time that he came to me. Genuine Stammering was his trouble, and so it was diagnosed. He refused to admit that he had a severe case, although the truth of the matter was, he did stammer badly and the mental power which had sustained him in his attempts to speak, was being steadily weakened by what we might term misuse.

He placed himself for treatment, although in a frame of mind that did not augur well for his success, but by the end of the third day his mental attitude had entirely changed, he came to realize the immense difference between being able to speak fluently and naturally and being compelled to substitute synonyms. From that day forth he was one of my best students. His education stood him in good stead, his enthusiasm was so spontaneous as to be contagious and at the end of four and a half weeks, he departed, as thoroughly changed for the better as anyone could wish. The arrogance was gone. In its place was something better--a sure- footed confidence in his ability to talk--and this was a confidence based on real ability--not on bluff. He was no longer nervous and irritable--and in fact, before leaving, he had won his way into the hearts of his associates to the extent that all were sorry when he left and felt that they had made the acquaintance of a young man of remarkable power.

Five years later, I met him in New York, quite by accident. He was in charge of his father's business, had made a wonderful success of his work and was universally respected and admired by those who knew him. Even to this young man, who to many would have seemed to have all that he could desire, freedom of speech opened new and greater opportunities.

If I had the space to do so within the covers of one volume, I would gladly give many more cases, with description and diagnosis as well as results of treatment. Specific cases are always interesting, illuminating and conclusive. They show theory in practice and opinions backed by actual results.

But lack of space makes it impossible to give additional cases here. Those which have been given are typical cases--not the unusual ones. The out-of-the-ordinary cases have been avoided and the common types dwelt upon with the idea of "giving the greatest good to the greatest number."

Every reader of this volume who lives today under the constant handicap of a speech disorder, may well take new hope from the thought that "What man hath done, man can do"--again!

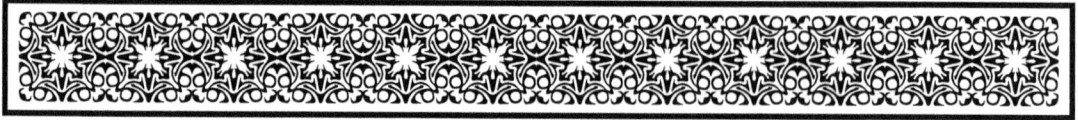

PART IV
SETTING THE TONGUE FREE

CHAPTER I
THE JOY OF PERFECT SPEECH

If you stammer--if you are afraid to try to talk for fear you will fail--if you are nervous, self-conscious and retiring because of your stammering--then you don't realize the Magic Power of Perfect Speech. You don't realize what perfect speech will mean to you. Listen to this--from a young woman who stammered--who was cured-- and who knows:

"The most wonderful thing has happened to me. What do you think it is! I have been cured of stammering. You have no idea how different it is to be able to talk. I just feel like I could fly I'm so happy. Just think, I can talk I'm so glad, so glad, so glad, it's over. I just feel like jumping up and down and shouting and telling everybody about it. I never was so happy in my life--I never was so glad about anything as I am about this."

That is the way she feels after being entirely freed from her stammering--after learning to talk freely and fluently without difficulty, hesitation or fear-of-failure.

And here are the words of a young man who has just found his speech: "The Bogue Cure is marvelous. It is just like making a blind man see. It is remarkable. The sensation of being able to talk after stammering for twenty-five years is wonderful."

And another young woman--this time from Missouri:

"That six weeks was the beginning of life for me. All my life I have had a dread of trying to speak which made life most unpleasant. I do not have it now--I love to meet people."

The joy of perfect speech:

The wonderful exhilaration of being able to say anything you want to say whenever you want to say, to whomsoever you desire to speak.

"I can talk"--that sums it all up. With that assurance comes the feeling of the innocent man freed from a long term in prison--the sense of completeness and wholeness and ability, the feeling that you are equal to others in every way, that you can compete with them and talk with them and associate with them on a plane of equality.

Such is the Joy of Perfect Speech!!

To know that the haunting fear is gone--that the shackles have fallen away, the chains are broken.

To know that you are free--delivered from bondage.

What a feeling--what a sensation--

Living itself is worth-while. Life means more. The sun shines brighter, the grass is greener, the flowers are more beautiful while friends and relatives seem closer, kinder and dearer than ever before.

The Joy of Perfect Speech!

No words can paint the picture, no tongue describe the lofty feeling of elation which crowns the man or woman or boy or girl who has stammered and has been set free.

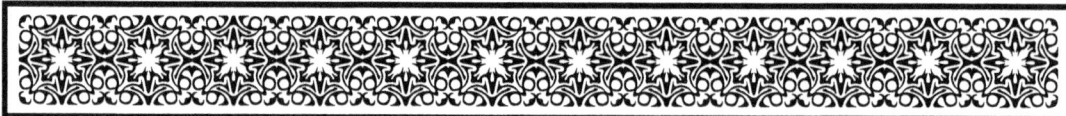

CHAPTER II
HOW TO DETERMINE WHETHER
YOU CAN BE CURED

You can either be cured of your trouble--or you cannot. If you can, why should you go about hesitating, stumbling, sticking, stammering and stuttering?

Why should you deny yourself the privileges of society, the advantages of opportunity, the fruits of success--if you can be completely and permanently cured of the trouble which handicaps you and holds you back?

Why should you live a HALF LIFE as a stammerer, if you can be cured and live the complete, joyous, happy, overflowing life?

Why should you be content with failure or half-success if the triumphant power to accomplish, the masterful will to succeed is right within your grasp?

Why should you continue to stammer if you can be cured?

The answer is, YOU SHOULD NOT.

The first step, therefore, is to determine definitely and accurately whether you are in a curable stage of your trouble and whether you can be completely and permanently cured.

These things you cannot determine for yourself. You have no facilities for determining the facts. You lack the scientific knowledge upon which such conclusions must be based. You cannot diagnose your case of stammering any more than you could accurately diagnose a highly complex nervous disease. In order, therefore, that the most important of all questions, viz.: "Can I be Cured?" may be correctly and authoritatively answered, I am willing to diagnose your case and give you a typewritten report of your condition, telling you whether or not you are still in a curable stage.

It goes without saying that this diagnosis must be based upon a description of the case in question. This description must be accurate and reliable as well as thorough. In order to insure this, I furnish with each book a Diagnosis Blank, which when properly filled out, gives me the information necessary to determine the durability of the case, as well as to furnish much other valuable information about the individual's condition.

In no case, will I undertake to pass on the curability of the stammerer without a diagnosis first being made. You want the opinion which I give you to be authoritative and dependable--a report in which you can place your entire confidence. I cannot give such a report by merely hazarding a guess as to your condition. I must base my report on the actual facts as they exist. I must make a careful study of your symptoms, determine what your peculiar combination of symptoms indicates, find out the nature of your trouble, determine its severity.

When you have returned the blank--and when I have furnished you with the diagnosis of your case, you can depend upon it to be accurate, authoritative, definite and positive. It will give you the plain facts about your trouble--be those facts good or bad.

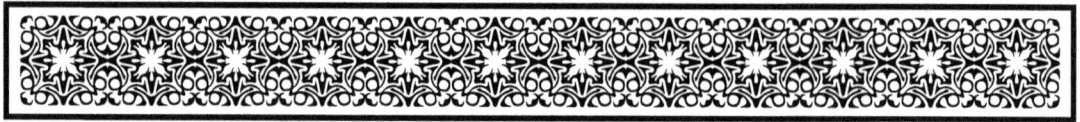

CHAPTER III
THE BOGUE GUARANTEE AND WHAT IT MEANS

No matter what caused your stammering, no matter how old you are, how long you have stammered, how many times you have tried to be cured--no matter what you think about your case or whether you believe it to be curable--if I have diagnosed your trouble and pronounced it curable, then I can cure YOU.

By the application of the Bogue Unit Method, I can eradicate the cause of your trouble at its very source, and re-establish normal co-ordination between your brain and the muscles of speech, removing every trace of that "mental expectancy" which you call "fear-of-failure."

I can show you how to place your articulation under perfect control, how to make the formation of words an easy process involving no apparent mental effort or noticeable physical exertion.

I can teach you how to produce any sound or combination of sounds, how to make every word an easy word and every sound an easy sound.

I can show you how to talk without stammering--how to talk just as freely and fluently as any normal person who has never stammered.

I not only claim to be able to do this for you, I back it up with a past record of success in treating hundreds of cases similar to your own. Like cures like. What has cured others like you, will cure YOU. But I don't ask you to risk a single penny upon even that evidence and proof. The moment you enroll in the Bogue Institute, I will issue to you and place in your hands, a written Guarantee Certificate, over my own signature, binding me to cure you of stammering or refund every cent of the money which you have paid me for tuition fee, and asking you only to follow the easy instructions given under the Bogue Unit Method.

You are to be the sole judge as to whether or not you follow instructions.

I will leave it entirely to you to decide. All I ask of you is full opportunity to do my best for you and absolute honesty, such as you expect and will receive from me.

I want to be absolutely fair with you--I want to cure you as I have cured myself and hundreds of other stammerers. I do not want a dollar of your money unless I have given you a dollar's worth of benefit in return. I would not keep a penny of the money that you might have paid me for cure of your stammering unless I had actually cured you, provided, of course, that you had followed the instructions which anybody of ordinary intelligence over eight years of age can easily follow.

I have no fear of your dealing dishonestly with me. I know enough about human nature to know that all you want is to be cured--and you understand that to be cured you must co-operate with me to that end. I can cure your stammering only with your co-operation-- just as a music teacher can make a pianist of you only with your co-operative and sincere effort. Therefore, I ask only that you follow my instructions carefully and faithfully--and I guarantee to bestow upon you the same gift of Perfect Speech that I have bestowed upon hundreds of now-happy men and women--and I put that guarantee in writing over my personal signature.

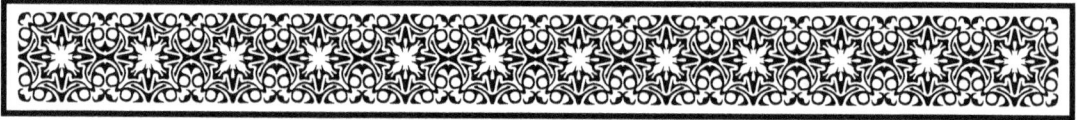

CHAPTER IV
THE CURE IS PERMANENT

No one who stammers should put any faith in a cure for his trouble unless the results are known to be permanent. A temporary cure is no cure at all and should be avoided, for it is merely a means of wasting money. The Bogue Unit Method brings about not only a complete but a permanent cure. The secret of its success as far as permanency is concerned, lies in the fact that the basic cause of the trouble is removed at its very source, the wrong methods rooted out and the correct methods installed in their place.

Once this process is completed and the cure effected, the cure is permanently insured, because its very cause is gone. You cannot stammer without a cause--everyone understands that.

The proof of the permanency of the cure is attested by the many letters from those who were here ten, fifteen, twenty years ago. A woman cured at the Institute ten years ago writes:

"At 14 I was a very bad stammerer. I then attended the Bogue Institute, where I was completely cured in a few weeks. I then secured a position as saleslady in one of our leading stores where I have been called upon to handle as many as one hundred sales in a single day. I have never stammered once. My cure has been absolutely perfect for the past ten years. It was certainly a lucky day that I walked into Mr. Bogue's office the first time."

Another excellent proof of the permanency of the cure, is the subjection of the cured student to tremendous mental and nervous strain. Many of our former students were in the Great War, numbers of them right up in the front line where the fighting was stiffest and where the nervous and mental strain was terrific. Even under this test (which was enough to make a normal person become a stammerer-

-and many of them did) the results of the Bogue Unit Method held them to normal speech. One young man writes:

"I completely regained my speech at the Bogue Institute in 1915. I enlisted in the army and was sent overseas in the spring of '18, and went through some of the hardest fighting the 42nd Division was in, that being the Division I was transferred to, and am happy to say the speech trouble has never come back on me. I was wounded by a fragment of high explosive shell. One hit me under the right arm, fracturing two ribs. Another struck my shoulder and a piece ranged downward into my right lung, which now remains there. I developed tuberculosis in November, in all probability from exposure as much as the wound. I was evacuated to the U.S. early last winter and sent to this place, where I am rapidly regaining my health and expect to be discharged about September 1st.

"With all the hard experience I went through, stammering did not come back to me. I have never regretted the time I spent with your Institute, and I have only the highest words of praise for the work being done in the Bogue Institute."

Another severe test of a cure of stammering is an illness such as may have brought the trouble on in the first place. If the stammerer, for instance, can undergo an attack of influenza or pneumonia and come out of it without difficulty, it proves beyond all question of a doubt that the cure is permanent.

For that reason, I wish to quote the letter of an Illinois boy who says:

"I am getting along fine with my speech. I am sure I will never stammer again. I was sick the week after Christmas with pneumonia but it did not bother me a bit."

Another young man says:

"It is now nearly six months since I left the Institute and in that time I have not stammered a word. What do you think about that? It surely is fine. But you know that. I was in Chicago last week and visited friends and saw a doctor friend of mine who did not know that I had been away, so he just stood there and looked at me, and said, 'You are talking fine. How did you learn that?'

"I told him and then talked to him for four hours and he said it was the best thing that had ever happened to me." Another letter, this time from Honolulu and from a man who attended the Institute a number of years ago, says:

"Just to let you know that I am still alive and enjoying life as I never have before. I have forgotten that I ever stammered. Sincere thanks to you."

This young man is now an engineer in the employ of the United Shipping Board.

These letters give the answer better than I can--better than any scientist can because they tell the real truth taken from the experience of those who have tried and know--

First--That stammering can be cured by the Bogue Unit Method!

Second--That the cure is a permanent cure!

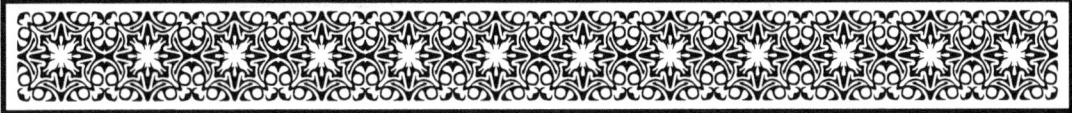

CHAPTER V
A PRICELESS GIFT--AN EVERLASTING INVESTMENT

There is no gift that can take the place of perfect speech. It is beyond price--and the person who talks after stammering would give all his possessions to keep from going back again to stammering.

But Freedom-of-Speech is more than a priceless gift--it is a wonderful investment. Should you ask: "Does it pay to be cured of stammering?" the answer could be nothing but "Yes"--and there is evidence aplenty to prove it.

One young man writes:

"I have never enjoyed life as I have since I left the Institute, both in a business and social way. I am to get a 25% increase in my salary the first of the month, which is at least partially due to my wonderful perfection of speech."

Does it pay--? Does a 25 per cent. increase in salary pay? Here is the case of a young woman who was about to lose her position because of her imperfection in speech--yet when she returned home after being cured at the Institute, she wrote:

"I was very much surprised when I went down to the office yesterday to find that I was going to get my place back again. This evening, Mr.--told me that I was to get a 33 1/3% raise at the end of next week, so my stay with you has already begun to pay dividends."

Freedom-from-Stammering PAYS--in dollars and cents. On a cold business basis, it is one of the best investments to be made. One man who attended here a few years ago was a fireman in a large factory, stoking boilers all day long. Today he is salesman--and the head salesman at that--for the same firm--he makes as much as the President of the firm. He works on commission--and he knows how to talk so as to sell.

Another man was section foreman when he took his course at the Bogue Institute. Today he is manager of one of a great chain of big retail stores and makes more in one day than he used to make in two weeks.

Another case is that of a young man from New York State, who gave up his position to come to the Bogue Institute and be free from stammering. Six weeks later he went home. Like the other young man mentioned above, he met with a success--surprise--he was re- employed by his old employers--and he, too, was given a 25 per cent. increase in salary.

So, you see, freedom from stammering pays--pays splendidly and continuously for all the rest of your life. It pays in satisfaction, in contentment, in happiness and ability to associate with others on a plane of speech-equality.

It pays in better salaries and bigger earning power--in opportunities opened and chances made possible to you that are closed to the one who stammers.

The world's successful men and women do not stammer. The happy, contented people do not stammer. The money-makers do not stumble and stick and stutter when they talk.

To be successful you must know how to talk. If you stammer today, make your plans to get out from under the handicap--remember that it will pay you and pay you well.

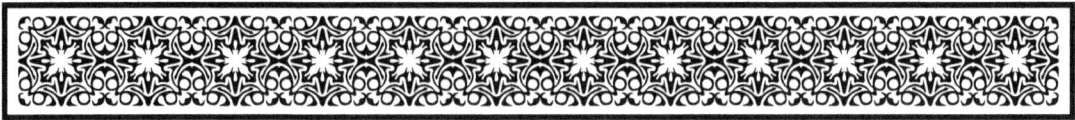

CHAPTER VI
THE HOME OF PERFECT SPEECH

The Bogue Institute of Indianapolis is truly the home of perfect speech. For in no other place can be found the things that are found here. Nowhere else is there that silent sympathy with the moods of the one who stammers. Nowhere else is there that home- like atmosphere, that all-prevading spirit of helpfulness and cheerfulness and good-will.

No matter how discouraged the stammerer may be, no matter how tired or nervous or self-conscious--no matter how shy or shrinking from the gaze of others--no matter how timid or filled-with-fear the mind, the attitude begins to change within an hour after his arrival.

For this is the home of perfect speech. Success is in the air. Every step I take counteracts the tendency to fear and worry and strain. I know what the stammerer needs. I know the things that need to be done to quiet the hyper-nervous case. I know what to do to banish that intense self-consciousness and make the student self-forgetful. These things have been learned by experience. And these gained-by-experience methods start the student in the right way from the very first hour.

Pupils Are Met at the Train: We are glad to meet pupils at the Union Station, where all trains over steam roads arrive, if the student informs us beforehand (either by letter or telegram) the road over which he is coming and the time he will arrive in this city. There is no charge for this, it being merely a part of the courtesy extended to students who are unfamiliar with the location of the Institute. A small bow of blue ribbon should be worn as a means of identification.

When You Arrive: If you have not written or telegraphed us to meet you at the railway station, as soon as you arrive go to the telephone booth and call the Bogue Institute and a representative of the institute will be sent for you promptly.

Your Baggage: The transfer of baggage from the station to the Institute will be attended to by our office. The Baggage Transfer makes regular trips to the Institute for the purpose of looking after the baggage of new students as well as those who have completed the course and are leaving for home.

Entrance Requirements: It is necessary that every student entering the Institute be of normal intelligence and at least eight years of age. Every student must also be of good moral character and must be able to speak the English language sufficiently well to take the instruction. When a stammerer has been cured in one language, however, he is cured in all languages. Rich and poor are here treated with equal kindness, courtesy and respect. We believe in those who are here to be cured, regardless of their station in life, and we believe in helping them accomplish that purpose in as short a time as is consistent with the results which they desire.

Grounds and Buildings: The Institute Building and Dormitory stand in a large lot, ideally located, in a desirable residential neighborhood away from the dirt, dust, noise and clamor of the city and yet not so far out as to be in the least removed from the city's activities.

Board and Room for Students: The Institute maintains its own Dormitory and Boarding Department under the direct and immediate supervision of the Institute authorities. To the right of the Main Dormitory Building as you enter will be found the Dormitory for girls and women, while on the left are located the General Offices and the Dormitory for boys and men. Every facility has been provided for the comfort and happiness of our pupils while at the Institute. Room, board, heat, light, hot and cold baths and all other comforts and conveniences are provided.

Sleeping Rooms: The pupils' sleeping rooms and apartments are large, well-lighted, and well-ventilated. They are comfortable both summer and winter, ample facilities being provided to heat the entire building comfortably at all times.

All of the sleeping rooms as well as the entire Dormitory and class-room are lighted with electricity. Each room contains furnishings necessary to make the room comfortable and home-like. Bath and face towels are furnished without extra cost, as is all necessary bedding and linen. Commodious and spacious bathrooms, with running water, and modern equipment are furnished for the exclusive use of pupils.

Dining Room: Two large, airy and well-ventilated dining rooms are located in the Main Dormitory Building. Here are served all meals, made up in the most appetizing manner--wholesome menus planned for the special needs of the type of students who come here. There is no dieting, but meals are carefully balanced and highly seasoned dishes or injurious food combinations are eliminated.

Every meal is prepared under the direct supervision of an experienced chef. Under this direction our pupils are served with some of the most delicious and healthful viands which can be put together--all of which is evidenced by the students' enthusiastic approbation of the Institute table fare.

Scrupulous Cleanliness: Every part of the Institute Buildings is kept scrupulously clean--every day in the year. In this respect the Bogue Institute surpasses many of the best hotels.

Library: The leading papers and magazines are constantly available and we encourage students to keep in touch with the world of events by regular reading.

How the Time is Spent: The order of the day is as follows:

6:30 AM	Arise
7 to 8 AM	Breakfast
8 to 9 AM	Special Study
9 to 11 AM	Morning Treatment Period
11 to 12 AM	Progress Tests, Special Examination and Personal Instruction
12 to 2 PM	Luncheon Period
2 to 4 PM	Class Instruction
4 to 6 PM	Recreation
6 PM	Dinner
8 PM	Children's Junior Class Retiring Hour
9 PM	Children's Senior Class Retiring Hour
10 PM	Adults' Last Retiring Hour

There are no classes on Saturday afternoon nor on Sundays or holidays. There are no evening or night classes at any time and no student may enroll who is not in a position to devote all the needed time to the pursuit of the work. There is no part-time course, permitting the student to work or go to public or high school while attending the Bogue Institute. The work here is too important to become a "side-issue." We insist that it be the student's regular and only absorbing activity.

LECTURES: From time to time during the year, open lectures are given by myself and assistant instructors dealing with the fundamentals of speech or kindred subjects aimed to make for the students' rapid progress. These lectures are important and must be attended by every student.

A CAREFULLY-PLANNED COURSE: Every step of the student's course from the time of arising in the morning to the time of retiring at night, is planned for the best results. Experience has taught us what is best and the day's program is built upon the lines of greatest progress in a given time. There are no haphazard steps in this program--each activity accomplishes a desirable and necessary result. These are the things that make for sure and rapid success --and which insure that every day shall show progress over the day before. In the work of the Bogue Institute every student's course is under my direct and personal supervision and direction. I am, of course, necessarily aided by assistant instructors, each of whom was selected with especial reference to his fitness for the work which is entrusted to him.

Every Teacher is a Specialist: Each one is a specialist--a master, backed not only by a thorough experience in the Bogue Institute, but also having served an extended apprenticeship under my personal instruction. Every specialist responsible for any department of our instruction must meet certain rigid qualifications. First, they must be well- educated, refined and of the best character. They must understand the stammerer's difficulty from a moral and mental standpoint as well as from a technical standpoint. They must maintain a naturally sympathetic, cheerful and helpful frame of mind at all times and must be able to prove that the training under my hand has thoroughly qualified them to serve the pupils of the Bogue Institute.

The long period of training and apprenticeship, which has always been an outstanding feature of our methods, could be done away with, should I desire to cheapen the instruction. Inexperienced instructors could be employed for less than half the compensation of the experts I now employ--but these things could be sacrificed only at the expense of results. For many years the superiority of the Bogue Institute faculty has been nationally recognized and this reputation we are today maintaining--and improving, where this is possible.

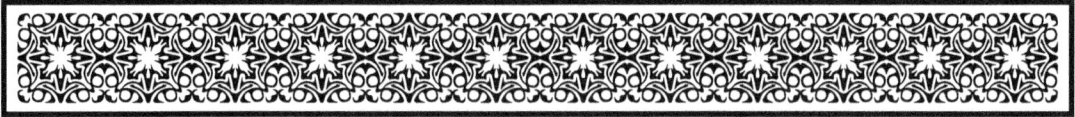

CHAPTER VII
MY MOTHER AND THE HOME LIFE
AT THE INSTITUTE

The home life at the Bogue Institute cannot be mentioned without also mentioning my mother and the work she has done and is doing to make this truly a home life. This is her work and she has succeeded. She represents the pivotal point around which that home life turns and she is the guiding spirit that makes the Institute a real home for those who come here. It is her beneficent smile that makes you feel at home when you arrive, her kindly influence which makes you feel at home during your whole stay and her smiling God-speed when you go, that makes you wish it were not time to leave.

Under Mother Bogue's direction, the Institute is a busy, happy, cheerful and well-ordered home for the big and happy family that it houses.

Music is here for those who wish to play. Games and books and magazines for those who would thus entertain themselves and others. We are acquainted with the truth that "all work makes Jack a dull boy--and Jill a dull girl"--and wholesome and worth-while amusements and diversions are provided for all ages and all occasions. These amusements are for those who wish them--those who do not can always find rest and quiet in their own rooms.

Rowdyism is absent. The hoodlum is not here. We find no difficulty in establishing standards of conduct that become the lady and the gentleman--and the regulations that are in effect are based upon the belief that those who come here can and will measure up to these standards.

Unity of Purpose: One of the distinct advantages of the plan whereby all students live in the Institute Dormitory is that all who are here have come for a purpose and bear that thought in mind. The student who sits beside you at the table is here for the same purpose as yourself. You are both working for the same thing --working earnestly, enthusiastically, seriously--and withal, successfully--to be cured of stammering.

What does this mean?

It means that the very atmosphere of the Institute is saturated with energy, enthusiasm and the spirit of successful endeavor. Determination, application, success--these things are in the very air you breathe. The spirit that carries an army to victory is here--to carry you to victory and success.

Absolute Privacy in Treatment: There is absolutely no publicity connected with the attendance of any student at the Institute. Many students have attended without even their families or friends being aware of the fact. Others have come leaving behind the impression that they were visiting friends--which in truth, they were, as they afterwards found those connected with the Institute to be sincere and worth-while friends, indeed.

Even in carrying on correspondence regarding the course, no one need know anything about your intentions, for upon no occasion does the name of the Institute appear on the outside of any letter or package addressed to you. Only the name "BENJAMIN N. BOGUE" appears to identify the letter.

At no time will your name, address or any information about you in connection with your name be published or discussed in any public manner whatsoever without your permission.

Care of the Health: Every safeguard is thrown around the physical welfare of those attending the Institute. The location and extraordinary sanitary precautions almost preclude the possibility of protracted illness--this was evidenced by the startling fact that during the severe and nation-wide influenza epidemic of the fall and winter of 1918-1919, not a single student of the Institute was taken ill. This speaks wonders for the remarkable good physical condition of the many students who were here at that time.

In the event, however, that a student does become ill, the Institute House Physician is at once summoned and in the case of a child, this physician's opinion will be sent immediately to the parents.

In illness as in health, the kindly, courteous and yet unobtrusive services of

Mother Bogue are at the disposal of the student. Every care is bestowed, special meals provided and every want looked after with the same pains as if the student were in his or her own home.

Christian Influences: Indianapolis is a city of numerous beautiful churches of all denominations, many of which are in the immediate vicinity of the Institute. During the entire stay, students are surrounded by the very best moral and religious influences and each Sunday sees groups of students leaving the Institute to attend services at the different churches.

Children Properly Cared For: Children placed in our care are given special attention. As with the other students they are surrounded with the most wholesome moral influences. Regulations provide that they must remain inside the Institute grounds except during the proper hours of the day, following their regular work. It is a very frequent occurrence to have parents bring their children with the idea of remaining with them during the course, only to return home within a few days, leaving the children with us, having satisfied themselves in that short time that the children are being just as well cared for here as if they were in their own homes.

Parents sometimes remark that children will get homesick and want to go home, but our experience with hundreds of cases proves that it is usually the parent who gets homesick to see the child instead of the child getting homesick to see the parents. The home-like surroundings of the Institute and the care and attention which they are given, allow small opportunity for children to become homesick, especially when it is remembered that they are busy for the larger portion of the day, at work which is to them of absorbing interest. In fact, we often find that children make so many good friends that they are reluctant indeed when the time comes for them to return home. Many of our students can testify that some of the finest friendships of their lives had their beginning here at the Bogue Institute.

Care for Ladies: My lady-assistants, as well as Mother Bogue, will see to the comfort and enjoyment of lady-pupils. Ladies have their own dormitories in a separate portion of the building and find their stay a most enjoyable one.

A Reflection of Ideals: The congenial home-life at the Institute, the minute attention to the wants of the students, the care given to women and children, the solicitude for those who are ill or who for any reason need special attention--this is but the reflection of an ideal--that ideal is to make the Bogue Institute, not only in instruction and results, but in every way, just what I would have liked to have been able to find when I was searching for a cure for stammering, more than twenty-five years ago. The comforts, the conveniences, the atmosphere of helpfulness--these things all contribute toward your quick and certain success--and that, I may say, is why we have them.

THINGS YOU WANT TO KNOW

Deposit Surplus Money: As a matter of convenience to those who bring with them extra money, we grant them the privilege of depositing it in our safe. Other valuables may be left for safe- keeping when desired. If the students prefer, they may deposit money with one of the city banks. Pupils should not carry much money with them; they may lose it.

Pupils' Mail: Relatives, friends and others addressing letters to persons in attendance at this Institute should address all mail to students: "c/o BENJ. N. BOGUE" to avoid delay in delivery.

Foreign Students: It will be necessary for those who speak foreign languages to learn the English language before they will be admitted to this Institute. The instruction is only given in English, but persons of all nationalities can be cured if they have the proper knowledge of the English language. When once cured in one language, persons are cured in all languages, however.

Companions for Pupils: Parents, guardians or companions may accompany small children or others, when they wish to do so. It is entirely satisfactory for those accompanying the pupil to be associated with the children during treatment. They may room together, if desired, or they may secure adjoining rooms.

When You Leave for Home: When necessary, we secure railroad tickets for our young pupils, check their baggage and place them safely aboard the proper train, when they leave Indianapolis for home, and otherwise take especial and careful interest in having them properly started homeward after their stay with us.

Rich and Poor Stand Equal: Claim is made that this is one of the most commendable features of the Institute. It is not so in all institutes. Fine clothes and freedom with money are not the test by which the student secures his standing, but by his earnest, faithful work and gentlemanly or lady-like conduct. It is inward worth, not outward adornment and display of wealth, that wins friends and gives the student a place on our roll of honor. The student is judged by what he is, and not by what he has.

Neglected Education: No one need hesitate to place himself under our instruction on account of neglected education or advanced age. All embarrassments are carefully avoided. Scores of backward pupils, who do not even know how to read or write, enter every year, and are entirely and permanently cured by the Unit Method.

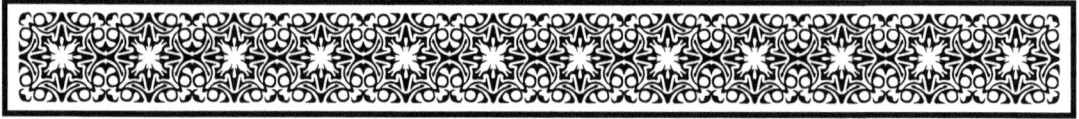

CHAPTER VIII
A HEART-TO-HEART TALK WITH PARENTS

If you are the mother or father of a child who stammers, you should first of all read Chapters IX to XIV, inclusive, in Part Two of this book. These chapters deal with the speech disorders of children from before the first spoken word up until the age of 21, when structurally as well as legally the mind and body of the infant merge into that of the adult.

No mother or father can understand their child's disorder without having read these Chapters. To fail to understand is to multiply the chance for error in deciding what to do. Therefore, I repeat, if you are the mother or father of a boy or girl who stammers, read chapters on Child Stammering before you go further.

There are three mistaken beliefs in the minds of many parents of stammering children which must be rooted out before the child will have an opportunity to be cured of his trouble.

These beliefs are:

    1--That the child will outgrow his trouble and therefore need
        only be permitted to "grow older," at which tune the trouble
        will disappear.

    2--That the child could stop stammering if he would try--that
        the trouble is but a malicious habit of the child's, which
        he could put away from him if he would.

    3--That the child's trouble is incurable and that nothing can
        be done for him.

All of these beliefs are entirely fallacious and based purely upon ignorance of the cause and progress of the child's trouble. There is not the slightest scientific foundation for them, they are not beliefs based on facts or upon experience--yet in many homes, they constitute the chief obstacle between the stammering child and his complete and permanent cure.

As long as you believe that your child will out-grow his or her trouble, you take no steps to have the disorder eradicated.

What happens?

The trouble becomes worse from month to month and from year to year, until in many cases where the "outgrowing belief" persists, the trouble passes into a chronic and incurable stage and the stammering child becomes the stammering man or woman, condemned to go through life under a handicap almost too great to bear.

Write it on your heart that your child will not outgrow his trouble. Ponder over the information given in the Chapters on Child Stammering. This is not hearsay or guess-work but facts gleaned from a lifetime of experience.

If you, as the father or mother of a stammering child, cling to the second belief, that your child could stop stammering if he would try, then I can see from this distance that your child has stored up for him in the future, more than his due of misery. For as long as you believe that he can stop of his own free will, you will be impatient with him when he stammers. You will scold him and tell him to "stop that kind of talking!" Thus you will irritate him, and bring to his heart that sickening sensation that he is totally helpless in the grip of his speech disorder and yet-- "Oh, why will they not understand?"

Like the first belief, this belief that the child could stop if he wanted to, is based upon ignorance. No mother or father who has ever experienced the sensation of fear that grips the heart of the stammering child when he tries to speak, will say that he could stop if he would.

I say to you--and I want to emphasize this--that the first and foremost ambition of your child who stammers, is to be free from it. The greatest day of his life will be the day when he can talk without that fear, without sticking and stumbling and hesitating over his utterances.

I say to you again--if that boy or girl of yours could stop their stammering, he or she would stop it this very instant. They would never stammer again--if they were endowed with the power to stop. But they are not. That is the very seed of their trouble--their inability to control the actions of the vocal organs so as to produce normal speech. They have lost the control of those organs and they cannot of their own volition re-establish that control.

The third belief, that stammering cannot be cured, is so easily demolished that I shall devote but little time to it. It, like all false beliefs, has its foundation in ignorance. The mother or father who knows the facts, knows also that stammering can be cured. You may not know whether your boy or girl can be cured, but you are offered a way to find out--definitely and positively, by describing your child's case on my Diagnosis Blank and returning it to me for a thorough Diagnosis.

Put your beliefs to one side--whatever they may be. You can get the facts if you want them. You can learn the truth if you will. Truth is better than false beliefs and facts are better than superstition or hearsay, which in every case leads to misery, dejection and despair--a ruined life where a successful, happy and contented life might have been--except for stammering.

You have a well-defined responsibility to your son or daughter. You have a duty to perform--that is, to equip that boy or girl of yours to go out into the world as well equipped as any other boy or girl--and that means equipped with perfect speech--without which they will be too greatly handicapped to fully succeed.

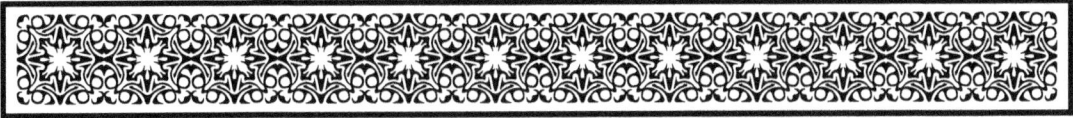

CHAPTER IX
THE DANGERS OF DELAY

In many of the cases which have come to my attention in the past many years, the stammerer or stutterer has been afflicted with a malady more difficult to cure than stammering, viz.: The Habit of Procrastination.

"Oh, I will wait a little while," says the stammerer. "A little while can't make any difference!" And then the little while grows into a big while and the big while grows into a year and the year grows into a lifetime and he is still stammering.

Several months ago, an old man, stooped in stature, care-worn of countenance and halting of step, presented himself to me for diagnosis. His face was drawn into long, hard lines. His eyes shifted from side to side, glancing furtively here and there.

In his trembling hands was a worn old derby which he turned about nervously as he stood there talking. The nervousness, the trembling of the hands, the drawn face, the shifting eyes--all this was explained by the story that this man told as he sat there beside the desk.

"I fell from a ladder when I was ten years old," he said. "After that, I always stammered. My parents thought it was a habit--I can remember yet how my mother scolded me day after day and told me to 'quit talking that way.' But it was useless to tell me to quit. I COULDN'T quit! If I could have done it, certainly I WOULD, for having stammered yourself, you know what it means.

"School now began to be a burden. I think I must have supplied fun for every boy on the school grounds during recess-time, for if there was a boy who didn't make fun of me and mock me and laugh at me, then I don't know who he was.

"Then one day I started back to school at noontime, saw a crowd of boys on the corner a couple of blocks away, thought of what a task it would be to go into that crowd or try to pass it. A mortal and unreasoning fear came over me. Try as I would, I couldn't screw my courage up to the point of going past that crowd. But I had small choice. It was either go that way or stay out of school. And stay out of school I did.

"And then came the crucial day. I could not ask my parents to vouch for any absence--I dared not tell them I was not there. So I went back without an excuse. The teacher was angry. She tried to get me to talk, but I could not say a word. So she sent me to the principal. She, too, asked me to explain. Try as I would, I couldn't get the first word out. Not a sound.

"She, too, failed to understand. Result: I was expelled from school--sorry day--nobody seemed to understand my trouble--nobody seemed to sympathize with me--a stammerer.

"Although I pretended to be at school, before the week was out, my parents found out. Then a storm ensued. I tried to tell them the truth. They wouldn't listen. Father stormed and mother scolded. There seemed to be no living for me there. So I ran away from home--ran away because my parents wouldn't listen--because they wouldn't try to understand.

"Then my troubles began in real earnest. I won't worry you with the details. I got a job--lost it. Got another--lost that. How many times that story was repeated I do not know. And remember--I was but a boy!"

Here the old man stopped, his head dropped, his unkempt beard brushed the front of a tattered shirt, that had seen its day. He seemed lost in thought--he was living again those days and those nights when he had wandered an outcast from the world. He was living over a lifetime in a moment.

He sat there several moments--thoughts far away. Then he raised his head and there was a tear in the corner of his eye as he said, "But why should I go on? Look at me. See WHERE I am. See WHAT I am. You would think I am over 70--I am not yet 50. But it is too late to do any good. Here I am homeless, friendless, almost penniless. Nobody cares what happens. Nobody would notice if anything should happen. Nobody has a job for me--a stammerer. If I could talk, I could work. If I could talk--Oh, but why tell it again? It is too late now--too late to do any good!!"

He was right. It was too late. Too late, indeed.

This man was one of the Too-Laters--one of the Put-It-Offs, one of the Procrastinators. His might be called the story of the Man Who Waited.

First, his parents refused to listen. His teachers, even, failed to understand his trouble. And when he got out in the world he put it off, this matter of being cured of stammering. He Waited! He kept saying to himself that he would do it tomorrow--next week-- next month. And tomorrow never came. Next week and next month ran into next year--and next year ran into a case that was hopeless and incurable.

He Waited!! How tragic those two words. He Waited! And his waiting sounded the death-knell of a thousand boyhood hopes. HE WAITED!! And health slowly took wings and flew away. HE WAITED!! And the insidious little Devil-of-Fear piece by piece tore down his will- power, sapped his power-of-concentration. HE WAITED!! And that first simple nervous condition turned into something near akin to palsy.

On the tombstone of that man when they lay him under his six-feet- of-earth, they might truly inscribe the words: "A Failure"--and should they wish to set down the reason, they might add: "He Waited!"

To the stammerer's question: "When should I begin treatment for my stammering?" and "At what stage will I stand the best chance of being most quickly cured?" there is but one answer. The time for the stammerer or stutterer to begin treatment for his malady is the day he discovers his stammering or stuttering. The best chance for being quickly cured exists today.

The stammerer, then, to paraphrase Emerson, should "Write it on his heart that TODAY is the very best day in the year." He should remember that indecision, delay, uncertainty, vacillation, lead to oblivion and that his only redemption lies in that golden opportunity known as--TODAY!

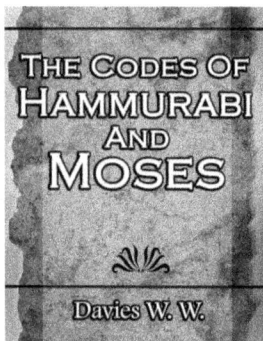

The Codes Of Hammurabi And Moses
W. W. Davies

QTY

The discovery of the Hammurabi Code is one of the greatest achievements of archaeology, and is of paramount interest, not only to the student of the Bible, but also to all those interested in ancient history...

Religion   **ISBN: *1-59462-338-4***   **Pages:132**
MSRP $12.95

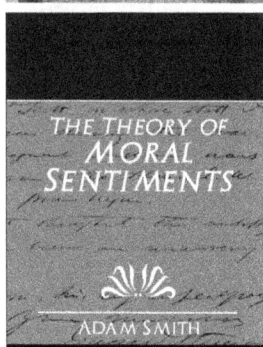

The Theory of Moral Sentiments
Adam Smith

QTY

This work from 1749. contains original theories of conscience amd moral judgment and it is the foundation for systemof morals.

Philosophy ISBN: *1-59462-777-0*   **Pages:536**
MSRP $19.95

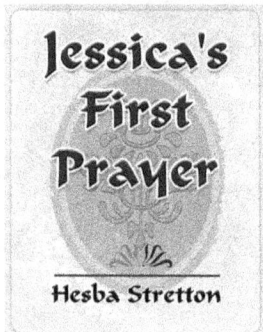

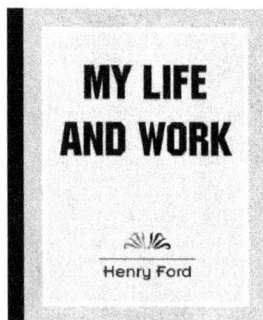

Jessica's First Prayer
Hesba Stretton

QTY

In a screened and secluded corner of one of the many railway-bridges which span the streets of London there could be seen a few years ago, from five o'clock every morning until half past eight, a tidily set-out coffee-stall, consisting of a trestle and board, upon which stood two large tin cans, with a small fire of charcoal burning under each so as to keep the coffee boiling during the early hours of the morning when the work-people were thronging into the city on their way to their daily toil...

Pages:84

Childrens   ISBN: *1-59462-373-2*   *MSRP $9.95*

My Life and Work
Henry Ford

QTY

Henry Ford revolutionized the world with his implementation of mass production for the Model T automobile. Gain valuable business insight into his life and work with his own auto-biography... "We have only started on our development of our country we have not as yet, with all our talk of wonderful progress, done more than scratch the surface. The progress has been wonderful enough but..."

Pages:300

Biographies/   ISBN: *1-59462-198-5*   *MSRP $21.95*

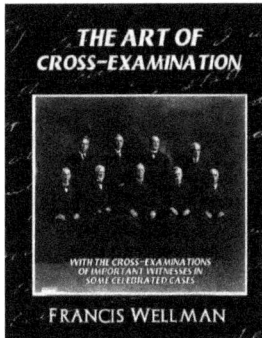

The Art of Cross-Examination
Francis Wellman

QTY

I presume it is the experience of every author, after his first book is published upon an important subject, to be almost overwhelmed with a wealth of ideas and illustrations which could readily have been included in his book, and which to his own mind, at least, seem to make a second edition inevitable. Such certainly was the case with me; and when the first edition had reached its sixth impression in five months, I rejoiced to learn that it seemed to my publishers that the book had met with a sufficiently favorable reception to justify a second and considerably enlarged edition. ..

Pages:412

Reference   **ISBN: *1-59462-647-2***   *MSRP $19.95*

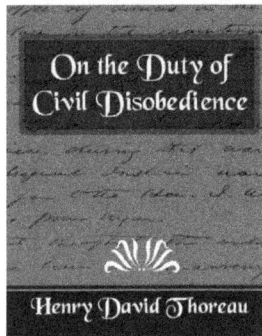

On the Duty of Civil Disobedience
Henry David Thoreau

QTY

Thoreau wrote his famous essay, On the Duty of Civil Disobedience, as a protest against an unjust but popular war and the immoral but popular institution of slave-owning. He did more than write—he declined to pay his taxes, and was hauled off to gaol in consequence. Who can say how much this refusal of his hastened the end of the war and of slavery ?

Law   **ISBN: *1-59462-747-9***   **Pages:48**
MSRP $7.45

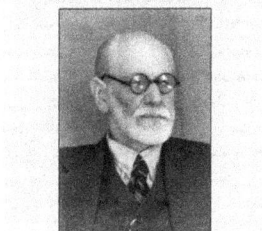

Dream Psychology Psychoanalysis for Beginners
Sigmund Freud

QTY

Sigmund Freud, born Sigismund Schlomo Freud (May 6, 1856 - September 23, 1939), was a Jewish-Austrian neurologist and psychiatrist who co-founded the psychoanalytic school of psychology. Freud is best known for his theories of the unconscious mind, especially involving the mechanism of repression; his redefinition of sexual desire as mobile and directed towards a wide variety of objects; and his therapeutic techniques, especially his understanding of transference in the therapeutic relationship and the presumed value of dreams as sources of insight into unconscious desires.

Pages:196

Psychology   **ISBN: *1-59462-905-6***   *MSRP $15.45*

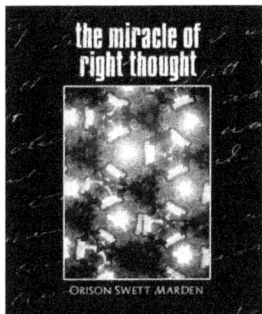

The Miracle of Right Thought
Orison Swett Marden

QTY

Believe with all of your heart that you will do what you were made to do. When the mind has once formed the habit of holding cheerful, happy, prosperous pictures, it will not be easy to form the opposite habit. It does not matter how improbable or how far away this realization may see, or how dark the prospects may be, if we visualize them as best we can, as vividly as possible, hold tenaciously to them and vigorously struggle to attain them, they will gradually become actualized, realized in the life. But a desire, a longing without endeavor, a yearning abandoned or held indifferently will vanish without realization.

Pages:360

Self Help   **ISBN: *1-59462-644-8***   *MSRP $25.45*

QTY

The Rosicrucian Cosmo-Conception Mystic Christianity by *Max Heindel*   ISBN: *1-59462-188-8*   **$38.95**
The Rosicrucian Cosmo-conception is not dogmatic, neither does it appeal to any other authority than the reason of the student. It is: not controversial, but is: sent forth in the, hope that it may help to clear...   New Age/Religion Pages 646

Abandonment To Divine Providence by *Jean-Pierre de Caussade*   ISBN: *1-59462-228-0*   **$25.95**
"The Rev. Jean Pierre de Caussade was one of the most remarkable spiritual writers of the Society of Jesus in France in the 18th Century. His death took place at Toulouse in 1751. His works have gone through many editions and have been republished...   Inspirational/Religion Pages 400

Mental Chemistry by *Charles Haanel*   ISBN: *1-59462-192-6*   **$23.95**
Mental Chemistry allows the change of material conditions by combining and appropriately utilizing the power of the mind. Much like applied chemistry creates something new and unique out of careful combinations of chemicals the mastery of mental chemistry...   New Age Pages 354

The Letters of Robert Browning and Elizabeth Barret Barrett 1845-1846 vol II   ISBN: *1-59462-193-4*   **$35.95**
by *Robert Browning* and *Elizabeth Barrett*   Biographies Pages 596

Gleanings In Genesis (volume I) by *Arthur W. Pink*   ISBN: *1-59462-130-6*   **$27.45**
Appropriately has Genesis been termed "the seed plot of the Bible" for in it we have, in germ form, almost all of the great doctrines which are afterwards fully developed in the books of Scripture which follow...   Religion/Inspirational Pages 420

The Master Key by *L. W. de Laurence*   ISBN: *1-59462-001-6*   **$30.95**
In no branch of human knowledge has there been a more lively increase of the spirit of research during the past few years than in the study of Psychology, Concentration and Mental Discipline. The requests for authentic lessons in Thought Control, Mental Discipline and...   New Age/Business Pages 422

The Lesser Key Of Solomon Goetia by *L. W. de Laurence*   ISBN: *1-59462-092-X*   **$9.95**
This translation of the first book of the "Lemegton" which is now for the first time made accessible to students of Talismanic Magic was done, after careful collation and edition, from numerous Ancient Manuscripts in Hebrew, Latin, and French...   New Age/Occult Pages 92

Rubaiyat Of Omar Khayyam by *Edward Fitzgerald*   ISBN:*1-59462-332-5*   **$13.95**
Edward Fitzgerald, whom the world has already learned, in spite of his own efforts to remain within the shadow of anonymity, to look upon as one of the rarest poets of the century, was born at Bredfield, in Suffolk, on the 31st of March, 1809. He was the third son of John Purcell...   Music Pages 172

Ancient Law by *Henry Maine*   ISBN: *1-59462-128-4*   **$29.95**
The chief object of the following pages is to indicate some of the earliest ideas of mankind, as they are reflected in Ancient Law, and to point out the relation of those ideas to modern thought.   Religiom/History Pages 452

Far-Away Stories by *William J. Locke*   ISBN: *1-59462-129-2*   **$19.45**
"Good wine needs no bush, but a collection of mixed vintages does. And this book is just such a collection. Some of the stories I do not want to remain buried for ever in the museum files of dead magazine-numbers an author's not unpardonable vanity..."   Fiction Pages 272

Life of David Crockett by *David Crockett*   ISBN: *1-59462-250-7*   **$27.45**
"Colonel David Crockett was one of the most remarkable men of the times in which he lived. Born in humble life, but gifted with a strong will, an indomitable courage, and unremitting perseverance...   Biographies/New Age Pages 424

Lip-Reading by *Edward Nitchie*   ISBN: *1-59462-206-X*   **$25.95**
Edward B. Nitchie, founder of the New York School for the Hard of Hearing, now the Nitchie School of Lip-Reading, Inc, wrote "LIP-READING Principles and Practice". The development and perfecting of this meritorious work on lip-reading was an undertaking...   How-to Pages 400

A Handbook of Suggestive Therapeutics, Applied Hypnotism, Psychic Science   ISBN: *1-59462-214-0*   **$24.95**
by *Henry Munro*   Health/New Age/Health/Self-help Pages 376

A Doll's House: and Two Other Plays by *Henrik Ibsen*   ISBN: *1-59462-112-8*   **$19.95**
Henrik Ibsen created this classic when in revolutionary 1848 Rome. Introducing some striking concepts in playwriting for the realist genre, this play has been studied the world over.   Fiction/Classics/Plays 308

The Light of Asia by *sir Edwin Arnold*   ISBN: *1-59462-204-3*   **$13.95**
In this poetic masterpiece, Edwin Arnold describes the life and teachings of Buddha. The man who was to become known as Buddha to the world was born as Prince Gautama of India but he rejected the worldly riches and abandoned the reigns of power when...   Religion/History/Biographies Pages 170

The Complete Works of Guy de Maupassant by *Guy de Maupassant*   ISBN: *1-59462-157-8*   **$16.95**
"For days and days, nights and nights, I had dreamed of that first kiss which was to consecrate our engagement, and I knew not on what spot I should put my lips..."   Fiction/Classics Pages 240

The Art of Cross-Examination by *Francis L. Wellman*   ISBN: *1-59462-309-0*   **$26.95**
Written by a renowned trial lawyer, Wellman imparts his experience and uses case studies to explain how to use psychology to extract desired information through questioning.   How-to/Science/Reference Pages 408

Answered or Unanswered? by *Louisa Vaughan*   ISBN: *1-59462-248-5*   **$10.95**
Miracles of Faith in China   Religion Pages 112

The Edinburgh Lectures on Mental Science (1909) by *Thomas*   ISBN: *1-59462-008-3*   **$11.95**
This book contains the substance of a course of lectures recently given by the writer in the Queen Street Hall, Edinburgh. Its purpose is to indicate the Natural Principles governing the relation between Mental Action and Material Conditions...   New Age/Psychology Pages 148

Ayesha by *H. Rider Haggard*   ISBN: *1-59462-301-5*   **$24.95**
Verily and indeed it is the unexpected that happens! Probably if there was one person upon the earth from whom the Editor of this, and of a certain previous history, did not expect to hear again...   Classics Pages 380

Ayala's Angel by *Anthony Trollope*   ISBN: *1-59462-352-X*   **$29.95**
The two girls were both pretty, but Lucy who was twenty-one who supposed to be simple and comparatively unattractive, whereas Ayala was credited, as her Bombwhat romantic name might show, with poetic charm and a taste for romance. Ayala when her father died was nineteen...   Fiction Pages 484

The American Commonwealth by *James Bryce*   ISBN: *1-59462-286-8*   **$34.45**
An interpretation of American democratic political theory. It examines political mechanics and society from the perspective of Scotsman James Bryce   Politics Pages 572

Stories of the Pilgrims by *Margaret P. Pumphrey*   ISBN: *1-59462-116-0*   **$17.95**
This book explores pilgrims religious oppression in England as well as their escape to Holland and eventual crossing to America on the Mayflower, and their early days in New England...   History Pages 268

www.bookjungle.com *email: sales@bookjungle.com fax: 630-214-0564 mail: Book Jungle PO Box 2226 Champaign, IL 61825*

QTY

The Fasting Cure by *Sinclair Upton*   ISBN: *1-59462-222-1*   **$13.95**
In the Cosmopolitan Magazine for May, 1910, and in the Contemporary Review (London) for April, 1910, I published an article dealing with my experiences in fasting. I have written a great many magazine articles, but never one which attracted so much attention... New Age/Self Help/Health Pages 164

Hebrew Astrology by *Sepharial*   ISBN: *1-59462-308-2*   **$13.45**
In these days of advanced thinking it is a matter of common observation that we have left many of the old landmarks behind and that we are now pressing forward to greater heights and to a wider horizon than that which represented the mind-content of our progenitors... Astrology Pages 144

Thought Vibration or The Law of Attraction in the Thought World   ISBN: *1-59462-127-6*   **$12.95**
by *William Walker Atkinson*   *Psychology/Religion Pages 144*

Optimism by *Helen Keller*   ISBN: *1-59462-108-X*   **$15.95**
Helen Keller was blind, deaf, and mute since 19 months old, yet famously learned how to overcome these handicaps, communicate with the world, and spread her lectures promoting optimism. An inspiring read for everyone... Biographies/Inspirational Pages 84

Sara Crewe by *Frances Burnett*   ISBN: *1-59462-360-0*   **$9.45**
In the first place, Miss Minchin lived in London. Her home was a large, dull, tall one, in a large, dull square, where all the houses were alike, and all the sparrows were alike, and where all the door-knockers made the same heavy sound... Childrens/Classic Pages 88

The Autobiography of Benjamin Franklin by *Benjamin Franklin*   ISBN: *1-59462-135-7*   **$24.95**
The Autobiography of Benjamin Franklin has probably been more extensively read than any other American historical work, and no other book of its kind has had such ups and downs of fortune. Franklin lived for many years in England, where he was agent... Biographies/History Pages 332

Name	
Email	
Telephone	
Address	
City, State ZIP	

☐ **Credit Card**   ☐ **Check / Money Order**

Credit Card Number	
Expiration Date	
Signature	

Please Mail to: Book Jungle
PO Box 2226
Champaign, IL 61825
or Fax to: 630-214-0564

ORDERING INFORMATION

web*: www.bookjungle.com*
email*: sales@bookjungle.com*
fax*: 630-214-0564*
mail*: Book Jungle PO Box 2226 Champaign, IL 61825*
or PayPal *to sales@bookjungle.com*

Please contact us for bulk discounts

DIRECT-ORDER TERMS

**20% Discount if You Order
Two or More Books**
Free Domestic Shipping!
Accepted: Master Card, Visa,
Discover, American Express